DISCOVER THE TRUTH ABOUT MIGRAINE MYTHS

Myth: Having migraines is a sign that you have psychological problems.

Fact: Migraine is a biological disorder, not a psychological symptom. In some people the period before a migraine is accompanied by mood changes, including irritability and depression. These are a result of temporary biochemical changes in the brain, not a permanent mood disorder.

Myth: A particular type of person tends to get migraine: hypersensitive, uptight, perfectionist, compulsive.

Fact: Researchers who have intensively studied the personality makeups of migraineurs have found no evidence of a "migraine personality."

Myth: You bring migraines on yourself. It's all in your head.

Fact: Migraine is a genuine medical disorder—as real as heart disease, high blood pressure, or diabetes.

Myth: There isn't much you can do about migraine; you just have to learn to live with it.

Fact: Migraine can't be cured, but in most cases it *can* be controlled. Research over the last decade has found effective treatments, including methods to prevent attacks or lessen their frequency.

NOW DISCOVER WHAT YOU CAN DO TO
RELIEVE YOUR SUFFERING.

MIGRAINE: THE COMPLETE GUIDE

MIGRAINE:

THE COMPLETE GUIDE

THE AMERICAN COUNCIL
FOR HEADACHE EDUCATION

with
Lynne M. Constantine
and Suzanne Scott

A Dell Trade Paperback

A DELL TRADE PAPERBACK

Published by
Dell Publishing
a division of
Bantam Doubleday Dell Publishing Group, Inc.
1540 Broadway
New York, New York 10036

The ideas, procedures, and suggestions in this book are not intended as a substitute for the medical advice of a trained health professional. All matters regarding your health require medical supervision. Consult your physician before adopting the suggestions in this book, as well as about any condition that may require diagnosis or medical attention. For information about proper use of the medications discussed in this book, talk to your physician. The authors and publisher disclaim any liability arising directly or indirectly from the use of this book.

The cases and examples cited in this book are based on actual situations and real people, and the personal statements quoted were drawn from interviews conducted for this book. Names and/or identifying details have been changed to protect privacy.

Library of Congress Cataloging in Publication Data

Migraine : the complete guide / by the American Council for Headache
    Education and Lynne M. Constantine and Suzanne Scott.
        p.   cm.
    Includes bibliographical references and index.
    ISBN 0-440-50458-9
    1. Migraine. I. Constantine, Lynne M. II. Scott, Suzanne.
III. American Council for Headache Education.
RC392.M615   1994
616.8'57—dc20   93-27843
                                                    CIP

Printed in the United States of America

Published simultaneously in Canada

May 1994

10

To Michelle,
Elizabeth, Billy,
Stephanie, David, and
the millions of other
migraine survivors whose courage
and perseverance inspire our work.

Contents

Acknowledgments

Completing a book of this scope requires the help and support of many people. In particular the authors wish to thank the following:

Physician members of the American Council for Headache Education, who contributed their clinical and scientific knowledge and provided careful and thorough critiques of the manuscript at every stage. Special thanks go to Joel Saper, M.D.; Fred D. Sheftell, M.D.; J. Keith Campbell, M.D.; Neil H. Raskin, M.D.; Seymour Solomon, M.D.; and Ninan T. Mathew, M.D.

Linda Hayes of Columbia Literary Associates, who developed the idea for the project, brought all of us together to make it happen, kept the project on track throughout the writing process, and infused the manuscript with her deeply lived knowledge of how migraine affects people's lives.

Robert K. Talley, Executive Director of the American Association for the Study of Headache, and Christine O'Keefe, former

Assistant Director of the American Council for Headache Education, who assisted in many ways great and small throughout the project.

Nancy Ginn Almond, former editor of the *ACHE Newsletter*, who provided advice, encouragement, and a wealth of information about migraine and migraineurs.

Catherine Avery, who assisted with the interviews for the book and provided encouragement and valuable advice during the writing process.

Marcia Seawell of the Rocky Mountain Headache Association, who was our host during a public information meeting co-sponsored by RMHA and ACHE in Denver, Colorado, and who graciously arranged for us to meet with a group of migraineurs who participate in RMHA support groups.

Ruth and Bill Ragsdale of the Florida Headache Association, who were generous with their time and information, particularly about setting up headache support groups.

Our families, who were supportive of the project from its inception and who shared our enthusiasm as it took shape.

And a special thank-you to the migraineurs who use the CompuServe® and Prodigy® on-line information services, to the many Rocky Mountain Headache Association members who participated in group and individual interviews, and to the dozens of other people throughout the country who were kind enough to share their stories with us for use in this book. Every paragraph of this book was written with you in mind. We hope you are pleased with the result.

Foreword

As many as 23 million Americans—approximately one in five women and one in twenty men—experience migraine, a painful and often disabling headache disorder. As a physician who has spent nearly two decades treating people with migraine, I have witnessed the enormous impact this condition has on these people, their families, and society. Yet no condition of such magnitude is more shrouded in myth, misinformation, or mistreatment.

Despite the fact that headache is the seventh leading reason for consulting a physician, many people seeking help for migraine have been shunted down a corridor of endless diagnostic procedures, ineffective treatment, and unfulfilled promises.

Millions and millions of dollars are wasted and additional suffering inflicted needlessly through inappropriate and unnecessary treatment. As a result of these encounters with well-meaning but ill-informed practitioners, patients with migraine and other headache disorders have found themselves with worsened headache and with treatment-related illnesses, including surgical complications, addictive disease, and drug toxicities resulting in liver, kidney, or gastrointestinal damage. They have been sent for nasal and sinus surgery, jaw reconstruction, hysterectomy, neck surgery, allergy shots, hormonal manipulation, myotherapy, and physical therapy. Every diagnostic tool in the modern medical armamentarium has been tried in the hope of finding something to fix or remove.

The irony is that, for patients with migraine, there is nothing to find and nothing to fix. Migraine is a chronic condition, like diabetes, heart disease, and hypertension. It reflects disturbances in the brain that are primary processes. And while headache can be controlled and effectively treated, the underlying disorder will be present for decades or even throughout the patient's life.

The misunderstandings and mistreatment result in much confusion and despair among patients and their families. Because a medical model for headache has been lacking, migraine patients have experienced discrimination and repudiation by insurance carriers and employers, and have been stereotyped and stigmatized by even the best-intentioned physicians, family members, and friends. These patients radically alter their lives to accommodate periods of headache-induced debility, believing that their only choice is to live with their head pain. Often they also harbor the self-defeating belief that their pain is "all in their head," because a physician has implied that their headaches are psychological in origin.

Added to these basic misunderstandings are the costs of unnecessary and often harmful treatments. Whether reckoned in money, in time, or in squandered hopes, these costs are immeasurable.

Typically, it is only after years of needless suffering that someone with difficult-to-treat headaches encounters a physician with a fundamental understanding of the disorder. Many patients who consult me have become addicted to painkillers over the years, but it is clear to me that they are not, for the most part, deliberate substance "abusers." They are the survivors of treatment failure, desperately seeking ways to carry on when their physicians neither understand nor can help.

But there is cause for optimism. Headache is emerging to join the ranks of what society accepts as legitimate illness. The medical community has demonstrated a commitment to understanding and treating this pervasive and disabling condition, as shown by growing interest in the work of the American Association for the Study of Headache (AASH) and the enthusiastic response to the formation of the American Council for Headache Education (ACHE).

My colleagues in AASH and I share considerable excitement over new research confirming our view that brain disturbances and chemical changes cause headache. This new information will prompt the development of new treatments for migraine and other headache disorders and will lead to more effective use of current treatments.

I hope we can also put to rest the erroneous but common belief that headache, and particularly migraine, is primarily caused by emotional distress. Asthma, epilepsy, schizophrenia, Tourette's syndrome, autism, Alzheimer's disease, obsessive-compulsive disorders, and manic-depressive disease all were once believed to be emotional in origin. The development of research-based medical models for these conditions, however, has considerably lessened the stigma and misunderstanding associated with them.

The members of AASH founded ACHE so our patients will have access to reliable information about migraine and other headache disorders and their treatment. Through our public education efforts we also hope to change societal attitudes, so that no one will have to experience stigma and self-doubt because of a brain abnormality and its resulting symptoms.

We are still far from reaching that day, but I believe people with migraine have many reasons to take heart. Today they can find physicians who recognize that migraine is a legitimate and at times disabling condition that is not caused by stress or personality flaws or by a patient's parents. And in a growing number of cities across the U.S., they can find active support groups in which people with migraine share their experiences and help each other feel less ashamed and alone.

It should no longer be an embarrassment to have a headache. People with migraine deserve our respect and support, as well as the best efforts of the medical and research communities to alleviate their pain.

—Joel R. Saper, M.D., FACP
Director, Michigan Headache
and Neurological Institute
National Chairman, American Council
for Headache Education

Introduction

If you or someone you love is among the millions of people who experience migraine headaches, you may feel that migraine controls your existence. This book is an invitation to take back that control and move on to a more satisfying life.

Migraine: The Complete Guide is an authoritative source of information, support, and practical help for anyone who suffers from migraine. It is based on the best information available: the findings of medical research, the clinical experience of leading experts on migraine, and the personal stories of dozens of migraine sufferers interviewed specifically for this book. It is a comprehensive resource to help you understand the illness of migraine and find effective treatment.

If you follow the recommendations in this book, you can almost certainly look forward to a future with fewer migraine attacks, a reduced intensity of attacks, and lessened fear that a headache will disable you without warning or recourse.

Far too many people believe they have to learn to "live with" migraine. They try to tough out the debilitating pain, the hours or days spent lying in the dark, the "uh-oh" feeling when the warning symptoms of impending headache appear, and the uneasy sense that others consider them malingerers or self-coddling hypochondriacs.

Far too many people blame themselves for their headaches. They believe headaches are "caused" by eating, working, or living wrong. When they get headaches on the job, they may be ashamed because they think it means they can't take the pressure. When they get migraines at home, they may fear disrupting the family's plans or facing unsympathetic responses from their spouses or children.

No one should have to feel shame or guilt about migraine and the disruption it creates. People do *not* cause their own headaches. Migraine is an illness—an inherited biological abnormality of the central nervous system. Migraine attacks result from changes in brain physiology. The mood changes, sleep disturbances, and other symptoms that accompany the attack arise from the same biological abnormalities.

For this reason migraine is far more than just a headache. It is a complex physical syndrome that may affect vision, thinking, and the functioning of many organ systems throughout the body.

This new understanding of migraine is the result of more than two decades of research and clinical experience by physicians specializing in headache. Their work shows that 85 to 90 percent or more of all migraine sufferers can hope to find significant relief with currently available treatments if they receive appropriate help.

The process of finding the right help, however, is not always easy. It takes time for new knowledge to become fully integrated into the everyday practice of medicine. Some physicians still do not take recurrent headaches seriously enough. Others, although they may be well-meaning and sympathetic, may not be familiar enough with recent research on migraine to diagnose and treat it properly. Even those who are up-to-the-minute in their approach to the disorder may not have spent enough time explaining the treatment process to you, so you may have stopped treatment prematurely when the first attempt to help you failed.

With migraine, as with any chronic illness, nothing is more important than developing a strong working partnership with a supportive physician. The key to this doctor-patient partnership is *knowledge:* both you and your doctor must be willing to learn as much as you can about migraine disorder. Knowledge will help you understand the unique patterns of your migraine attacks, communicate that information to your doctor, participate intelligently in your treatment, evaluate the treatment you receive, and ask for additional help if you're not seeing significant improvement.

This book has been created to give you the knowledge you need. We have divided it into three parts so you can easily find answers to your most pressing questions about migraine.

In Part One, "Understanding Migraine," you will find a complete overview of what science knows about migraine: the causes, the triggering factors, who gets migraine, and how a typical migraine attack presents itself. Understanding what happens to you during an attack will go a long way toward dispelling the fear and panic you may feel about your headaches. It will also prepare you to map your unique migraine profile, so you can communicate your experience of migraine to your doctor.

Part Two, "Treatment for Migraine," contains a comprehensive review of the medical and nonmedical ways to relieve and prevent migraine attacks. From diagnosis to self-care, these chapters focus on what you, the patient, need to know to take control of your migraines. You will discover what treatments are available and how to find the ones that are right for you. You'll also learn how to take care of yourself, avoid factors that seem to trigger your headaches, and talk to your doctor about your responses to treatment.

In Part Three, "Living with Migraine," you'll find a wealth of practical advice for living well with migraine. You'll learn techniques for educating employers, teachers, family, and friends;

ways to cope with migraine on the job; essential information to make sure your child isn't shortchanged at school just because she or he has headaches; traveling tips for migraine sufferers; and ideas for coping with the effects of migraine on your family.

Migraine is not a disgrace, a curse, a judgment, or a sign of personality problems. It is a treatable illness. We hope that by reading this book you will become more confident that you *can* take control of your headaches.

PART ONE

Understanding Migraine

CHAPTER 1

What Is Migraine?

"Everyone thinks I'm being dramatic when I say I'd rather give birth to my children again than have a migraine. I'm not. My headaches hurt worse than childbirth."

"They say people with migraine have a lower suicide rate than the rest of the population. It's not because we wouldn't do it. Most of us would cheerfully kill ourselves during an attack, but we're just too sick."

"I've traveled a lot. My husband has great memories of Russia, China, the Grand Canyon, and so on. My travel memories consist mostly of vomiting in strange toilets."

Migraine is one of the most painful and frustrating benign disorders known to medicine. Migraine is considered medically "benign" because it is almost never life threatening or a direct cause of someone's death. But to a person who experiences migraine (often referred to as a *migraineur*), migraine is pernicious, evil, soul stealing, life robbing, expensive, exhausting, and humiliating. Measured by its effect on a migraineur's life, migraine is anything *but* benign.

Sit with a group of people who experience migraine headaches, and as you listen to them talk about their disorder, you'll notice a telling fact: the word they use most often for "getting a headache" is "die."

"I woke up yesterday morning and knew that the minute I'd move, I'd die."

"I was on the road fifteen minutes and started feeling like I was getting a headache, so I stopped at a motel and died."

The most extraordinary fact of all is that migraineurs, who frequently experience the most exquisite agony imaginable, look just like anyone else. Even when a headache is coming on, many force themselves to continue functioning normally for as long as possible, until they are overcome by the nausea, head pain, fatigue, and weakness that characterize migraine.

Unfortunately, their bravery and mettle backfire on them. Since there's no outward sign of their suffering—no broken bones, no gaping wounds, no perceptible disabling condition—sympathy from others can be hard to come by. Many people who don't experience migraine believe migraineurs are overdramatizing their pain or are malingering or looking for attention.

"It's just a headache," they say. "Take a couple of aspirins." Or, "It's probably allergies, it'll go away." If the person with migraine is a woman (and as many as three out of four are), she may hear, "Maybe you just can't handle pressure." Unfortunately, the physicians that migraineurs consult often have demonstrated similar attitudes.

In response migraineurs have hidden their condition all the

more. The result is a catch-22 that has left them feeling guilty, ashamed, confused, and despairing of ever finding any treatment to help them. They may wonder if they are, in fact, somehow responsible for their condition. Maybe it is "all in their head"!

AN ILLNESS, NOT A SYMPTOM

If you have migraines, it is time to forget every negative word or insinuation you've ever heard. Migraine is *real.* It's not something you are doing to yourself for any reason. You are having migraines because you have a physiological condition that predisposes you to these painful and often disabling headaches.

It is also important to recognize that migraine is more than "just a headache." The nausea, vomiting, sensitivity to light and sound, fatigue, weakness, irritability, vision problems, and other symptoms that accompany your headaches are an integral part of the migraine syndrome. Current research suggests that they are all part of the same biochemical process that causes migraine's characteristic head pain.

Migraine is what physicians call a "primary disorder." That is, it's an illness—not a symptom of something else that's wrong with you. Even if you have allergies, sinus problems, or mental health problems, they are not the causes of your headaches. From a medical standpoint the cause is in your body's chemistry, not "in your head."

Medical research still has a long way to go in figuring out the causes and specific mechanisms that give rise to migraine. What's already known, however, has led to a wide variety of new and promising treatments. Like arthritis or diabetes, migraine is a chronic condition, so it can't be "cured." But like other chronic conditions it can be managed and controlled.

WHAT DOES MIGRAINE FEEL LIKE?

At a recent conference for members of the American Association for the Study of Headache, the professional group for physicians who treat headache patients, a pharmaceutical company sponsored a special exhibit to try to replicate what migraine feels like. The display was in the form of a six-foot-tall head: you went into the head, sat down, pushed a button, and watched a video on migraine.

As you watched, a special light display inside the head demonstrated each stage of the migraine attack. First the lights simulated the unusual visual phenomenon, called *aura,* that precedes some people's migraines. As the aura faded, the light display on one side of the head grew brighter, pulsating rhythmically and insistently in time to the human heartbeat. By the end of the display people who had never experienced migraine felt lucky that they could walk away and know they'd never have to go through the real thing.

Even more dramatic, however, were displays of "migraine art" presented by several other drug companies. In these startling self-portraits, artists who have migraine headaches tried to convey their personal experience of pain. One artist depicted himself screaming in pain as a huge hand pulled his brain out through the top of his head. Another painted himself as lying helpless and naked on barbed wire while tiny blue creatures screwed his head into a vise, broke his forehead open with a pickax, and bored a needle into his eye. A female artist saw herself as a disembodied head skewered between two sharp wedges, with a fire raging inside her skull.

Migraine art is not a phenomenon of the late twentieth century. The original drawings for Lewis Carroll's classics, *Alice's Adventures in Wonderland* and *Through the Looking Glass,* may depict the phenomenon of aura. Carroll, who experienced severe migraines, is said to have directed the illustrator John Tenniel in these renderings.

Descriptions of the extraordinary pain associated with moderate to severe migraine go back as far as the Mesopotamian empire in 3000 B.C. The famed physician Hippocrates (460–357 B.C.) described the "violent pain" of what was surely a migraine episode. Another Greek physician, Aretaeus of Cappadocia (second century A.D.), noted the characteristic one-sided head pain of migraine as well as the "dreadful" accompanying symptoms.

The word *migraine* itself is a reference to the one-sided, throbbing head pain that many (but not all) people with migraine experience. The Greek physician Galen (A.D. 131–200) is credited with naming the headache *hemicranios,* which means "half-head." This word became *hemicranium* in Latin, *megrim* in Old English, and *migraine* in French and modern English.

The intensity of the pain of migraine is even harder to bear because it recurs so frequently—one to three times a month for the average migraineur. And the pain often lasts a long time. Most migraine headaches go on for at least four hours. Sometimes a single attack can continue for as long as seventy-two hours.

The presence of such extraordinary pain has led migraine patients and those who treat them to extremes in search of a cure. Purging, bleeding, tying a hangman's noose around the head, applying herbs to the scalp, and even trepanning (drilling a hole in the skull) all were tried as remedies. Pliny the Elder (A.D. 23–79), an eminent Roman who wrote a vast compendium of the natural sciences, scraped moss from the head of a statue and hung it by a string around the sufferer's neck. In our own day a variety of surgical procedures in and around the head and neck have replaced the arts of superstition—but often with as little scientific justification.

THE IMPACT OF MIGRAINE

The Denver-based Rocky Mountain Headache Association, one of the largest and oldest support organizations for people with headache in the U.S., and its sister organization, the Florida Headache Association, refer to headache as "the invisible handicap." The description is apt, because migraine can have the same profound emotional and financial impact as other disabilities.

Emotional Impact

> "It's hard for me not to feel like a failure as a mother. During the years my children needed me most, I would be completely out of commission about six or seven days a month. If I decided to barrel on through the pain, I'd wind up getting irritable with them. It breaks my heart to realize how much time they spent tiptoeing around, trying not to disturb me."

> "I can still see myself dressed up, smiling, greeting dinner guests, serving food, and disappearing to lie down for ten minutes or throw up. Then I'd return smiling until I had to disappear again."

Migraine takes an enormous toll on the quality of life for migraineurs and their families. "Migraine doesn't kill you outright, but it leaves huge holes in your life," said one woman. "It kills a little bit here and a little bit there."

Misinformation and misunderstanding about migraine can stress even the best relationships at home. Migraineurs may harbor years of secret hurt over the look on a spouse's face that unmistakably says, *Oh, no, not again!* Family members may feel angry and abandoned. "I recall a fight with my teenage daughter about something completely trivial, and in the middle she turned bright red and screamed at me, 'Why can't you be like other mothers and *not have headaches*!'" said one woman who experienced migraines for more than two decades.

At work migraineurs may feel the constant tension of having to meet job demands, never knowing when a headache will lay them low. They may come to work sick with a headache, fearful of losing their jobs because of too-frequent absences. "I finally decided to quit my job," said a woman who now is a full-time home-maker. "I just couldn't stand the anxiety."

Another woman decided to go into business for herself. "It's a lot better than working for someone else," she said, "but I know my assistant resents all the times she has to cover for me."

Over many years the guilt, shame, and frustration accompanying the recurrent attacks may result in depression, hopelessness, and an erosion of self-esteem. And as the last straw migraineurs are often mistakenly told that these *results* of their years of living with migraine are actually the *cause* of their headaches.

Financial Impact

Migraine has a profound effect on the financial well-being of migraineurs themselves, as well as on society as a whole. From a society-wide perspective headaches cost the nation more than $50 billion each year; half or more of this sum is attributable to migraine.

Migraine is a major contributor to lost productivity in the workplace. Migraineurs account for 92 million lost workdays each year, at a cost to the economy of over $11 billion. They also spend uncounted millions of days each year working at diminished productivity levels because of the severe head pain and visual and digestive disturbances.

Migraine also makes a significant contribution to this nation's health care costs. Few migraine-specific figures are available, but migraine probably accounts for half or more of the 50 million office visits per year attributable to headache. Migraine also accounts for a significant proportion of the $400 million spent each year for over-the-counter aspirin and other headache remedies, and for the millions more spent on prescription drugs for headache.

The societal cost of migraine takes on more meaning when you translate these national statistics into their potential impact on a migraineur's household income. The results can be truly staggering. "I can't say how many thousands of dollars I spent going from doctor to doctor before I finally got some real help," said one man. "And even now I'm still paying for it, because my health insurance premiums are astronomical."

CHAPTER 2

Myths About Migraine

"I never want people to know I have migraine—not so much because I'm afraid people will judge me, but because, in my secret soul, *I* judge me. I worry that there's something wrong with me. Maybe I just can't cope. Or maybe I'm looking for attention. I can tell myself it isn't true, but it eats away at me inside."

Recall, for a moment, the typical way you hear headache mentioned on television. The first image that probably comes to mind is one of the many commercials for headache remedies such as aspirin, acetaminophen, and ibuprofen. These over-the-counter pills are portrayed as miracle drugs that can banish even the toughest headaches in minutes.

Now consider the classic lines about headache in TV situation comedies. Who hasn't heard "Not tonight, I have a headache"? Or how about "I think I feel a headache coming on" when someone or something is causing stress?

And what about the medical dramas? Have you ever seen a kindly television doctor treat any type of headache?

Television programming and advertising reflect the myths we live by. And when it comes to migraine, the myths are pervasive, persistent, and highly destructive. If you have migraine, you probably believe many of the most common myths—*even though they directly contradict your own experience.* And if you, like many people with migraine, try to keep your illness hidden, you probably don't have a support group or informal network of fellow migraineurs who can help you do some "reality checking."

Separating fact from myth is the first step toward understanding migraine. If you're a migraineur, it also is the first step toward overcoming any guilt or shame you may feel about your condition.

REPLACING MYTHS WITH FACTS

Do any of the following seventeen myths about migraine sound familiar? Most of us, whether we have migraine or not, believe most of them without even thinking. Considered in the light of the latest scientific research, however, all these beliefs are nothing more than biases.

If you have taken any of these myths to heart, replace them with the corresponding facts. Changing erroneous beliefs in this way will help give you a new, more positive outlook on living with migraine.

MYTH: **Having migraines is a sign that you have psychological problems.**

FACT: Migraine is a biological disorder, not a psychological symptom. Migraineurs come in all shapes, sizes, and states of mental health. Some people with mental health problems may have migraine, but migraine is not the cause or the result of these problems. (For more on the causes of migraine, see Chapter 4.)

In some people the period before a migraine is accompanied by mood changes, including irritability and depression. These are a result of temporary biochemical changes in the brain, not a permanent mood disorder.

"In my experience most people with migraine are *more* optimistic and better balanced than the average person, when they're not having a headache," said a member of a headache support group who frequently speaks to community organizations. "It takes that kind of person to keep going in spite of the pain and debility."

MYTH: **A particular type of person tends to get migraine: hypersensitive, uptight, perfectionist, compulsive.**

FACT: Researchers who have intensively studied the personality makeups of migraineurs have found no evidence of a "migraine personality."

Some migraineurs who display these personality traits may have developed them as a reaction to their illness. They may feel a strong need to keep order around them because they never know when their lives will be disrupted by a migraine attack. (For more on coping with emotions, see Chapter 24.)

Some experts suggest that this myth may be perpetuated by physicians who resent the demands of patients whose illnesses they can't successfully treat.

MYTH: **You bring your migraines on yourself. It's all in your head.**

FACT: Migraine is a genuine medical disorder—as real as heart disease, high blood pressure, or diabetes.

As in the case of other chronic diseases, you can learn ways to cooperate with your body to help control the effects of migraine disorder, but this does not mean you are causing your migraine attacks. (See Chapter 10, "Your Part in the Treatment Process.")

MYTH: **There isn't much you can do about migraine; you just have to learn to live with it.**

FACT: This destructive myth keeps far too many people from getting effective treatment. Migraine can't be cured, but in most cases it *can* be controlled.

Research over the last decade has identified several routes of effective treatment, including some methods to help prevent attacks or lessen their frequency. (See Part Two, "Treatment for Migraine.")

MYTH: **Migraine is so awful that it's got to be a sign of something terribly wrong.**

FACT: All of the manifestations of migraine are a temporary response to a biochemical chain of events in the central nervous system. When the biochemical balance returns to normal, the symptoms subside. Rarely are there any permanent complications. That's why migraine is called a "benign" disorder.

For example, some people fear that migraine may bring on a stroke, especially since some of the symptoms (such as confusion, weakness of limbs, and problems with speech) may mimic those of a stroke. Migraine-related stroke does occur, but it is an extremely uncommon complication of migraine and tends to occur in people with a specific pattern of symptoms. (For more on migraine-related stroke, see Chapter 20, "Uncommon Complications of Migraine.")

MYTH: **Women "use" migraine headaches to get out of having sex.**

FACT: Sex or any form of physical activity makes a migraine-in-progress hurt more. A woman or man who avoids sex during a migraine episode isn't necessarily trying to avoid intimacy. He or she probably is trying, quite sensibly, to avoid pain.

The disruption of normal family relations, including sexual relations, can be a distressing part of living with migraine. Effective treatment can lessen the impact, as can improved communication about the disorder and creative problem-solving techniques. (See Chapter 25, "Migraine and Family Life.")

MYTH: **Sinus trouble causes migraine.**

FACT: Sinus infection rarely is the cause of chronic recurrent headaches of any type. Some people are misled by television advertisements for decongestants and nasal sprays. These ads imply that sinuses are a major cause of headache.

Acute sinusitis, an infection of the sinuses around the nose, does occur, especially after a head cold, and can cause head pain. It is easily diagnosed by a physician and responds quickly to antibiotics.

MYTH: **Migraine is just an excuse to leave work early or to miss work altogether.**

FACT: Migraine patients are not malingerers. They have a legitimate medical reason to take time off from work for treatment and recovery.

A migraineur may have to leave work suddenly or stay home during an attack because of the symptoms associated with migraine, especially vomiting or sensitivity to light, sound, and motion.

Many people with migraine make themselves miserable so as *not* to miss work. They'll stay at work while they're in excruciating pain or come to work when they're nauseated and tired. (For more on migraine at the office, see Chapter 27.)

MYTH: TMJ is the cause of a lot of migraines.

FACT: TMJ, a problem with the temporomandibular joint between the upper jaw and the skull, has little or nothing to do with the head pain most people with migraine experience.

Many leaders in the headache field believe the importance of TMJ as a cause of headache has been pushed out of proportion. Be sure that you seek a second opinion from a nonsurgical medical expert if TMJ surgery has been suggested as a way to relieve your head pain.

MYTH: **Migraines are due to allergies.**

FACT: Coincidence is the only link between allergies and migraines. Allergies and headaches are common occurrences; because some people have both, they assume there is a connection. If you do have both allergies and migraine, your allergy treatments won't necessarily help your headaches.

Another factor in the confusion is that some migraineurs experience relief for their headaches when they take decongestants for their allergies. This may occur because one effect of decongestants is to constrict blood vessels, including those involved in head pain.

MYTH: **The more medication you take for a migraine, the better you'll feel.**

FACT: Exceeding the recommended dose of any medication won't provide more relief. Instead it usually creates serious problems.

Some people, for example, think that the worse a headache is, the more aspirin (or acetaminophen or ibuprofen) they should take for it. Studies have shown, however, that three aspirin tablets give no more relief than one tablet. Taking them more often than recommended only succeeds in loading your body with more medication without providing any more relief.

Many people think that because a drug is sold over the counter, it isn't as dangerous as prescription medications. This idea also is a myth. Taking more than the recommended dose of any medication is a bad idea. Too much aspirin, acetaminophen, or ibuprofen can cause serious side effects, such as damage to the stomach, liver, or kidneys.

If someone is taking a pain reliever, even an over-the-counter one, more than three days a week, the pain reliever may actually be making the headache problem worse. This phenomenon is called "rebound headache." (See Chapter 21, "Medication Overuse and Rebound Headaches.")

MYTH: **Migraine is an adult illness; with children, headache usually is a symptom of more serious illness.**

FACT: Somewhere between 7 and 18 percent of children, both boys and girls, experience migraine. Migraine has been diagnosed conclusively in children as young as three; some researchers believe it may even begin in infancy. Even in children, headaches usually are not a sign of more serious illness. The incidence of brain tumors, for example, is very low in both children and adults, and recurring headache is seldom the first symptom.

Even though there is probably no hidden illness, it's a good idea to see a doctor promptly if headache disrupts a child's schoolwork or social life; if the headaches begin suddenly or change in nature or frequency; if they are accompanied by numbness, weakness, double vision, or difficulty in balancing; or if they are associated with fever and/or stiff neck. (For more information on migraine in children, see Chapter 18.)

MYTH: **Migraines are caused by stress. If you could just learn to relax and enjoy life, you wouldn't have migraines.**

FACT: Stress does not cause migraine. Any amount of stress in a person who does not have a susceptibility to migraine will not produce a migraine. However, in a person susceptible to migraine, stress may be one of many "triggers" that can result in an attack.

Some experts think a triggering factor activates a series of biochemical events that were ready to be fired off. The trigger is a factor (e.g., a food, an environmental condition such as the weather, a lifestyle habit such as smoking or erratic sleep patterns —see Chapter 6 for a complete list) to which the person is particularly sensitized and which provides the spark for the biochemical reaction.

Having this biochemical reaction doesn't mean a person can't cope well with stress. The physical events are in the brain's chemistry, not in the person's thought processes; these events don't have anything to do with coping skills.

Many people being treated for migraine become confused about the relationship between stress and migraine when they are taught biofeedback or relaxation techniques as a means of controlling their headaches. Again, these recommendations are not a judgment on you as a person. They are prescribed as a way to help your body deal better with its physical sensitization to certain environmental stresses. (For information on relaxation techniques, see Chapter 15, "Nondrug Therapies.")

MYTH: **Migraine is a woman's disease.**

FACT: Migraine is two to three times more common in women than men, but millions of men also have migraine. Among children migraine occurs with equal frequency in boys and girls.

The myth that migraine is a woman's disease is destructive, because it denies men access to health care and at the same time stigmatizes women. The hidden message of the myth is that migraine is not a disease but a complaint of hysterical and weak women—a moral failing instead of a public health problem. (For more information on migraine in men, see Chapter 19.)

MYTH: **Migraine is just a part of PMS.**

FACT: Even when a woman's migraines are closely timed to her menstrual cycle, migraine is not just one of the symptoms of the disorder known as premenstrual syndrome or PMS. Although some of the same hormonal activity may be responsible for both disorders, each probably is linked to a different set of biochemical changes resulting from that hormonal activity. (See Chapter 17, "Menstrual Migraine.")

MYTH: **Migraine headaches can't be all that bad; I've had headaches, and I've managed. These people must be overly sensitive to pain.**

FACT: While sensitivity to pain is different for each person, there is no scientific evidence to show that people with migraine are more sensitive to pain than other people.

Some people who have mild to moderate head pain from time to time confuse the pain of their headaches with the type of pain experienced by people with moderate to severe migraine. That's something like comparing the pain of a hangnail to the pain of having a fingernail torn off.

The experience of millions of people with migraine, who often say that migraine is the worst pain they've ever encountered, shouldn't be dismissed so lightly. Considering the intensity of their pain, many migraineurs have learned to be exceptionally stoic, carrying on many of the functions of everyday life despite a level of pain that would demolish someone experiencing it for the first time.

MYTH: **Migraine must be a sign of intelligence because so many famous scientists, artists, and writers have had it.**

FACT: Even though well-known people like Thomas Jefferson, Sigmund Freud, Frédéric Chopin, George Bernard Shaw, Virginia Woolf, and others have experienced migraines, studies have shown that migraine is a democratic illness. It strikes geniuses and ordinary intellects, educated and uneducated, social elite and social outcasts with about equal frequency. Some recent studies suggest that, in the United States, people with lower income levels are more likely to be diagnosed with migraine. (See Chapter 3, "Who Gets Migraine?")

Physicians Have Myths About Migraine Too

Physicians have their own set of myths about migraine. Common physician myths reflect centuries of inaccurate and incomplete information about the causes of migraine.

The emerging medical model for headache will eventually make these myths a thing of the past. They will be relegated to the same dustbin as the belief that evil spirits trapped in the skull cause headache—a belief that led many European, Asian, and Pacific cultures to drill holes in the skulls of people with chronic headaches to let the demons out.

PHYSICIAN MYTH #1:   **Migraine is difficult to diagnose.**

FACT: In the vast majority of patients migraine is easily diagnosed through the person's family history, medical history, and symptoms. Migraine headaches have distinctive characteristics that set them apart from other types of headaches. (See Chapter 7.)

PHYSICIAN MYTH #2:   **Treating migraine is routine and uninteresting.**

FACT: Once properly diagnosed, treating migraine is an interesting challenge because as many as 85 to 90 percent of all patients will respond to appropriate therapy. The challenge lies in selecting the therapy most appropriate for the patient, then monitoring both success and side effects to adjust the treatment as necessary.

PHYSICIAN MYTH #3:   **Patients with migraine are hard to work with.**

FACT: Not so, according to the physicians of the American Association for the Study of Headache (AASH), who work with migraineurs every day. When the physician is knowledgeable about migraine, he or she recognizes that treating a migraine patient is no different than treating any other chronically ill patient. Migraineurs, in fact, tend to be highly motivated people willing to make significant lifestyle changes to improve their headache status.

PHYSICIAN MYTH #4:   **Severe migraine can't be helped.**

FACT: While some patients will not respond to currently available therapies, the vast majority achieve significant relief that improves their quality of life. Patients who do not respond to primary-care interventions now have options for advanced care by headache specialists, headache clinics, and comprehensive headache centers.

CHAPTER 3

Who Gets Migraine?

"No one that I knew of in my family ever had migraine. So when I would get my worst headaches, I'd find myself thinking, *Nobody gets headaches like these. I'm a freak.*"

If there's any consolation in having migraine, it's that you can be sure you're not alone. Migraine is a common condition. All kinds of people experience it, but they may be hiding it so well that you may never realize it.

Migraine is sometimes called "the democratic disorder" because it does not discriminate by gender, class, age group, race, or ethnic group. No matter how you slice the population, no group has yet proven to be exempt. Migraine afflicts all personality types, all ages (even children), both sexes, and all socioeconomic classes.

HOW MANY PEOPLE HAVE MIGRAINE?

Dependable statistics about the prevalence of migraine are hard to come by. Until recently the number of people included in population studies of migraine has been very small, and studies often were limited to specific groups such as children, the elderly, or people who consult neurologists. In addition the diagnostic criteria for migraine and other types of headache have not been standardized until recently, making data from different studies hard to compare.

For this reason, you may see a wide variety of estimates quoted in books and newspaper articles. The figures typically range from a low of 8 million to a high of 50 million.

A recent national survey of more than twenty thousand people, published in the *Journal of the American Medical Association (JAMA),* estimated the total number of Americans who experience recurrent migraine episodes at 23 million, or about 9 percent of the population. This figure makes it clear that migraine is a common disorder and one deserving serious attention.

MIGRAINE BY GENDER

Migraine researchers generally agree that migraine is equally common among boys and girls before puberty. But beginning at puberty far more women than men experience migraine. The biological basis for the difference is not yet fully understood, although the hormone estrogen is suspected to be an important contributor. (See Chapter 4.)

What also isn't clear is exactly how large the "gender gap" in migraine really is. For example, studies have shown that among adults who consult a physician about their migraines, women outnumber men by 4 to 1. But this figure may not be a good indicator of the number of men with migraine. Men may simply be less likely to seek help for their headaches than women.

The *JAMA* study estimated that the ratio of female to male

migraineurs in the general population is actually somewhere between 3 to 1 and 2 to 1. Among all migraineurs twelve and older who participated in that study, women outnumbered men by 2.8 to 1; among migraineurs between the ages of forty and forty-five, the ratio of women to men was 3.3 to 1. Even after age sixty-five, when any hormonal predisposition in women would have been reduced or eliminated by menopause, the ratio of women to men still remained quite high, at 2.5 to 1.

Using the estimate that there are 23 million migraineurs in the U.S., a reasonable estimate might be that 5.8 million of the total are men and 17.2 million are women. In other words, about 6 percent of adult men and 17.6 percent of adult women in the U.S. experience migraine.

MIGRAINE BY AGE

The majority of people with migraine—both men and women—are between the ages of twenty and forty-five. Migraine is more common among thirty-five- to forty-year-olds than among any other age group.

But migraine is not exclusively an adult disorder. Between 7 and 18 percent of all children experience attacks. Toddlers as young as three have been definitively diagnosed with childhood migraine, and some researchers have found evidence that children may begin having headaches as early as six weeks after birth. (See Chapter 18, "Migraine in Children.")

Migraine also is well known to decline with age. Among men the prevalence of migraine begins to decrease in the thirties; among women, it begins to decrease in the late forties.

At What Age Does Migraine Begin?

More than half of those who have migraines as adults had their first attacks before they left their teens. Ninety percent will have their first attack by sometime in their thirties. Rarely does migraine begin after fifty.

In women the onset of migraine may be linked with major hormonal changes. Many women begin experiencing migraine at or around menarche, the beginning of their menstrual periods. About 10 percent of women migraineurs experience their first migraine after forty, perhaps in response to the hormonal changes associated with menopause.

Does Age of Onset Affect Duration or Cessation?

The age you were when your migraines began seems to have very little to do with when (or if) they cease to trouble you. Some studies suggest that many—but by no means all—migraineurs can look forward to a decreased frequency and intensity of migraine attacks after age fifty.

Children who have migraines seem more likely to "grow out of them" than adults. Nearly half of all children who experience migraines will stop having attacks sometime during adolescence. Another quarter will stop during their early adult years.

Women whose migraines are closely linked to their menstrual cycles may see their migraines temporarily disappear during pregnancy, although the opposite effect sometimes occurs. In the same way, some women may find that their migraines diminish or disappear with menopause, while others find they continue more or less unchanged. Supplemental hormones, whether in the form of estrogen replacement therapy during menopause or birth control pills, frequently cause an increase in the number of headaches. (See Chapter 17, "Menstrual Migraine.")

MIGRAINE BY RACE

Not much is known for certain about the racial distribution of migraine in the United States. The *JAMA* study found that migraine was less common among African Americans, especially African-American males, than among white Americans.

Although this finding may not be very reliable, the researchers thought it might suggest a true biologically based difference. As evidence they pointed to the fact that African Americans have a higher blood level of an enzyme that metabolizes tyramine, a chemical in foods like red wine and cheese that act as migraine triggers. (See Chapter 6.)

MIGRAINE BY SOCIOECONOMIC GROUP

The stereotype has long held that migraine is an illness of the middle and upper classes, not of the workingman and -woman. The *JAMA* study, however, presented the first evidence that migraine may be more prevalent among people of lower income in the U.S. In the study the likelihood of someone having migraine increased as his or her annual income decreased. The prevalence of migraine was more than 60 percent higher in the lowest income groups than in the highest.

Exactly why the results of this study turned up a statistic contrary to the data collected by physicians across the country and by other, smaller, studies is unclear. The researchers proposed several possible explanations. Since migraine is a disabling condition, people with migraine may "drift" down the ladder of economic well-being because the illness interferes with work or school. This phenomenon of economic drift is very common with other disabling conditions.

Another possible explanation is that people of higher incomes have access to better health care or may be exposed to fewer migraine triggers in their diet or environment.

HOW OFTEN DO MIGRAINEURS HAVE ATTACKS?

According to migraine experts migraine may occur as infrequently as one attack in a lifetime or as frequently as several times in the same week. The typical migraine patient, however, experiences one to three attacks per month.

People between the ages of twenty and fifty experience migraine attacks more frequently than either children or the elderly. In the *JAMA* study people with lower incomes appeared to have more frequent attacks than people with higher incomes.

HOW COMMON ARE DISABLING MIGRAINES?

Of the 23 million American migraineurs estimated by the *JAMA* researchers, approximately 11.6 million—or slightly more than half—reported that they experience headaches that make it impossible for them to work or carry on other activities of daily life while an attack is in progress. Of these, 8.7 million are women and 2.6 million are men.

HOW DO INTERNATIONAL STATISTICS COMPARE TO THOSE OF THE U.S.?

Industrialized countries such as Canada, Great Britain, and the countries of Western Europe report similar migraine rates to those of the U.S. For example, a recent study in Denmark found that, over their lifetimes, 13 percent of Danes experience migraine. A study in France estimated that 12 percent of people over age fifteen were migraineurs. And a Canadian study estimated that 16.5 percent of adult Canadians experience migraine.

Other countries either do not report statistics or have reported ones whose reliability is unknown. The People's Republic of China, for example, reports very low rates of migraine among their population. But it is not known whether these low rates are real or merely reflect different definitions of migraine than those in use by other nations.

CHAPTER 4

The Causes of Migraine

If scientists could study a living human brain during a migraine attack, if they could track every action of nerves, arteries, and veins and every biochemical change that takes place, they might be able to give us a definitive answer about the causes of migraine. Such a study, of course, is impossible. Similar studies in animals also are out of the question, because there is no way for us to know whether any animal species experiences migraine. Scientists therefore have to rely on indirect evidence in their quest to understand this mysterious illness.

Fortunately, medical science has made enormous advances in technology during the past few decades. New imaging techniques such as magnetic resonance imaging (MRI), positron-emission tomography (PET), single-photon emission computed tomography (SPECT), and transcranial Doppler (TCD), along with the well-known CT (computed tomography) scanning technology, have made it possible to study blood flow in the brain without the need for potentially dangerous dyes or blood-vessel punctures. In addition researchers have come to understand much more about the complex life of brain cells and about the biochemical processes involved in pain.

As a result many old ideas about migraine have been put to rest, and new theories have arisen to guide research on methods of treatment. While not yet giving us a definitive answer on the cause of migraine, these new theories already are being used to create a new generation of "designer" migraine drugs. (See Chapter 23, "The Future of Migraine Treatment.")

NEUROBIOLOGY AND MIGRAINE

Until recently scientists believed that migraine was a problem chiefly related to blood circulation. As someone with migraine that theory may make a lot of sense to you: during migraine attacks many people can feel the throbbing of blood vessels in the head in time to their heartbeats. Scientists also had made some studies of migraineurs' blood circulation and found that blood flow decreased in the brain during the aura of migraine, then increased afterward.

Combining this evidence scientists assumed that the ultimate source of the aura, pain, and other accompaniments of a migraine attack was a tightening or constriction of blood vessels in the brain, neck, or scalp, followed by a sudden dilation (opening) of the blood vessels to larger than their normal size. The reduction of blood to the brain during the constriction phase, they believed, caused the aura of classic migraine. When the blood vessels dilated, the rushing blood swelled the vessels and brought on the throbbing pain.

This theory sounds so plausible, so painfully like your experience, that you may be surprised to learn that scientists no longer believe it. True, changes in blood circulation *do* accompany migraine. But it has now become clear that these changes are the *results* of the migraine, not the cause.

Today the consensus is that migraine is a biochemical disorder within the brain, not a blood-vessel (vascular) disorder. For one thing, scientists haven't found any real proof that the blood vessels contract in the way the older theory predicted. Only a very small number of angiograms (X rays of blood vessels in the head) taken on people while a migraine attack was in progress demonstrate specific areas of narrowing in the brain's blood vessels. Also, scientists have noted that blood vessels in the head may swell at times other than during a migraine attack, without causing the throbbing head pain accompanying many people's migraines.

One prominent researcher uses an analogy to explain how this biochemical abnormality of the brain works to cause a migraine. The brain of a person susceptible to migraine, he says, is like a computer with one chip that's especially susceptible to electrical "noise" such as static, power surges, or radio interference. The computer runs fine until there is a "pop" of static. Then the "noisy chip" sends out an unexpected signal, which affects the other chips in the machine and makes the whole system go awry. The only way the person working at the computer knows any of this has happened is that an error message appears on the screen —or the system just stops working. Similarly, someone susceptible to migraine may go along just fine until something triggers the brain's abnormal chemistry, beginning a cascade of events that eventually results in head pain.

A POSSIBLE MIGRAINE SCENARIO

Scientists are not yet sure of how the neurological and biochemical events that lead to a migraine actually work. But here's one possibility.

Migraine starts with a susceptible person—someone who probably was born with a central nervous system preprimed to develop migraines. This predisposition takes the form of a hypersensitivity to certain types of stimuli. It can be "triggered" by exposure to different factors in the person's lifestyle or environment, including foods or beverages, chemicals, sunlight, fatigue, stress, and hormones. (See Chapter 6, "Migraine Triggers.")

When a susceptible person encounters a trigger, the trigger causes the hypothalamus (a part of the brain behind the eyes) to signal cells deep within the brain stem (the base of the brain). Both the hypothalamus and the brain stem are part of the complex system that controls involuntary processes such as breathing, digestion, blood circulation, and pain perception—processes that are basic to life.

Scientists don't know exactly what the hypothalamus is trying to say to the brain stem about the migraine trigger. But they have identified several chemicals involved in the communication process, including the chemical signals (neurotransmitters) *serotonin* and *noradrenaline.*

Serotonin is a neurochemical that has powerful effects on smooth muscle tissue and the digestive system and causes large blood vessels to contract. Changes in serotonin activity within the brain are believed to be involved in sleep disturbances, in depression, and perhaps in addictive disorders such as alcoholism.

During a migraine attack serotonin activity in the brain changes dramatically. The serotonin disturbances may partly account for the head pain, and may also be responsible for the nausea, vomiting, and mood changes that accompany migraine.

The neurochemical noradrenaline also plays a part in the making of a migraine. In people who have migraine with aura, changes in noradrenaline activity cause a slowdown of activity in certain cells in the part of the brain called the cortex. This depression of activity results in a reduction of blood flowing to that area of the brain—because the neurons in the area don't need as much blood as they normally do for their metabolic activities. These changes seem to result in the neurological phenomenon we call the aura of migraine. The depression spreads in a wave across the cortex, much the way some people's migraine aura seems to spread across their visual field.

Serotonin and noradrenaline are only two of the many chemicals believed to be related in some way to migraine. Others include dopamine, tyramine, histamine, and various other chemicals called *amines* that have effects on the blood vessels. One of the challenges of migraine research is to tease out the separate contributions of each of these chemicals, then pick the points in the process where treatment can be most effective.

THE ROLE OF THE PAIN-CONTROL SYSTEM

Many scientists believe that another reason migraine headaches hurt so much is that the migraine process affects the body's pain-control system. The pain-control system, located deep in the brain stem, governs your perception of how much something hurts, as well as your body's automatic responses to limit the damage caused by injury of any kind.

The pain-control system works with a group of natural pain-control chemicals, called *endorphins,* manufactured by your body. These chemicals are similar in many ways to opiates such as morphine and cocaine. Some people call endorphins "the body's own opiates." But the endorphins can't work properly unless neurotransmitters like serotonin are present in the body in the right amounts. One theory of why migraines hurt so much is that the process of making a migraine uses up the body's store of serotonin and other neurotransmitters.

Another possible contributing factor is a chemical called *bradykinin,* a powerful irritant that is chemically similar to wasp venom. Like a wasp sting, bradykinin causes inflammation: it lowers the body's pain threshold, making the site where it accumulates highly painful, and causes blood vessels at the site of injury to dilate. During a migraine attack bradykinin accumulates around arteries in the scalp and may account for the localized pain, scalp tenderness, and burning sensations many migraineurs experience.

THE ROLE OF FEMALE HORMONES

Because migraine affects so many more women than men after puberty, and because hormone-related events such as pregnancy, menopause, and the cycles of menstruation seem to influence the timing and frequency of a woman's migraines, scientists are fairly certain that changing levels of female hormones play a role in migraine. But exactly how these hormones work is a mystery.

One possible factor is that estrogen is a potent stimulator of chemicals called *prostaglandins,* which cause blood vessels to constrict or dilate and which play a part in the experience of pain.

A recent study, for example, found that women with menstrual migraine had lower levels than normal of a prostaglandin called PGI_2. A woman's levels of PGI_2 tend to be high during pregnancy—a time when women with menstrual migraine often see their headaches improve or disappear temporarily. PGI_2 levels also increase when people with migraine use beta-blockers—a common migraine-preventive medication.

As with serotonin, however, the interaction of estrogen and prostaglandins probably involves other abnormalities than mere differences in the levels of these chemicals. For example, women who experience true menstrual migraine (i.e., women who get migraine headaches only during their periods or up to two days before or three days after) experience changes in the way their blood cells respond to prostaglandins during their time of susceptibility to migraine.

The question of hormone involvement in migraine will probably turn out to be far more complicated than just the effects of estrogen on prostaglandins. The hormonal system is regulated by a complicated internal clock, with hormones whose main function is to tell the body when to make and release female hormones. We may find that some mechanism in this "hormone clock" plays a role in the development of migraine. It may take many years to say definitively why women's hormones make them more susceptible to migraine than men.

IS MIGRAINE A DISTINCT FORM
OF HEADACHE DISORDER?

Anyone who has experienced a migraine can distinguish it from other types of headache: it *feels* different. The throbbing pain, the nausea and vomiting, and especially the prodrome phenomena (aura, mood changes, food cravings, for example—see Chapter 5) all seem to indicate that migraine is a specific type of headache, different from all others.

Scientists, however, aren't so sure. In particular, many now suspect that migraine and "tension-type" headaches are part of the same biological process, even though the clinical symptoms differ. Here are the three most common theories on the subject:

- **The "headache types" theory:** This theory holds that, while all headaches may affect the same neurotransmitter systems and biochemical processes, each headache type has a unique set of causes and must be seen as a separate illness. Some scientists even argue that migraine with aura and migraine without aura are different entities.
- **The "evolutionary headache" (or "headache continuum") theory:** This theory holds that a person who may begin having intermittent migraine headaches will have a tendency to evolve toward having chronic daily headaches similar to tension-type headaches, usually with intermittent migraines as well. This may mean that the two headache types derive from the same biological sensitivity, or that the repeated migraine episodes somehow influence the person's biochemistry or physiology to develop in this way. In at least 50 percent of the migraine patients who develop chronic daily headache, overuse of symptom-relieving medications such as aspirin or prescription painkillers contributes to the development of this headache pattern, although the overuse probably began in response to a need for more frequent use of medication to cope with this evolutionary process.

- **The "single-disease" theory:** This theory holds that all headaches may share a common mechanism, probably related to the actions of serotonin.

Which view is correct? No one is sure. One clue may be that the drug sumatriptan, which was designed especially to treat migraine patients, has shown great success in treating cluster headaches—the type of headache that seems most distinct from migraine. (For more on cluster headaches, see Chapter 7.) Another clue is that people who get migraines often have lots of tension-type headaches, even if they do not develop chronic daily headache.

Scientists don't yet know how to interpret these clues. The good news, however, is that they don't have to have all the answers to be able to help most migraine patients.

IS MIGRAINE INHERITED?

Most headache researchers now believe that heredity plays a major role in the development of migraine. In clinical studies at least 60 percent of migraineurs report having close relatives with the same problem. Of that group more than half had a mother with migraine; 17 percent, a father; 17 percent, a sister; and 12 percent, a brother.

It is clear from these statistics that a predisposition to migraine is transmitted genetically. Scientists think migraine is what's called an "autosomal dominant disorder," in which a single parent with migraine can pass on a predisposition to the illness. Early studies suggest that a rare form of complicated migraine, called familial hemiplegic migraine, may be caused by a genetic defect on Chromosome 19 (one of the twenty-six strands of DNA in human cells).

Does everyone with a predisposition to migraine eventually have migraine headaches? At this time there is no way to know, because there is no test for susceptibility to migraine.

Although susceptibility to migraine is inherited, susceptibility to a specific trigger probably is not. Being susceptible to a specific trigger is the result of your body's becoming sensitized to that trigger. Your body learns to respond to the presence of that trigger with a biochemical chain-reaction that ultimately leads to migraine.

Sensitization is itself a complicated process. Sometimes your body becomes sensitive to something because you're around it a lot: for example, if you live in a damp basement apartment, you may become sensitive to mold. Or if you have ten cats, and they all sleep in your bedroom, you may become sensitive to cat dander. But sometimes a single exposure to a substance, such as a particular chemical, can cause a powerful sensitization. Or sometimes it may be a combination of factors that sensitizes you: for example, you may only be sensitive to wine when you're tired or when you drink it in the hot sun.

For this reason triggers tend to be highly individual, even within a family. One woman may get a headache every time she eats chocolate; her daughter, however, may have no trouble with chocolate but may experience a violent attack when exposed to cigarette smoke or to flickering fluorescent lights. Learning about your individual triggers is an important part of controlling your migraines. (See Chapter 6, "Migraine Triggers," and Chapter 10, "Your Part in the Treatment Process.")

There's one other complicating factor in this issue of genetics and triggers, and that's the case of someone who develops migraines after a head injury or other trauma, such as an invasive neurological test like a myelogram or angiogram. Do these people have a genetic predisposition to the disorder, or does the trauma itself somehow initiate the disorder?

It's tempting to believe that the trauma is a trigger, because only some people who develop headaches after trauma seem to develop *migraine* headaches. Not all posttraumatic headaches are throbbing and accompanied by nausea, like those many migraineurs; many are more like tension headaches—a dull, relentless pain like a tight band, or a feeling of pressure or pulling in the scalp, face, and eye region. And not all posttraumatic head-aches recur over a period of years; many will clear up, never to return, after a period of weeks or months.

The fact is that researchers just don't know the answer yet. The mystery of posttraumatic headache is just one of the many remaining mysteries of migraine, despite all the progress scientists have made in understanding this complicated disorder.

CHAPTER 5

Types of Migraine
and Characteristics
of the Migraine Attack

Although migraine is one of the most common headache disorders, it is by no means a simple illness. Migraine comes in two "flavors" and several varieties. And even though its most noticeable symptom is a painful headache, the headache is merely the end point of a cascade of biochemical events that have a wide range of effects on the body. (For more on the biochemical processes involved in migraine, see Chapter 4.) As a result migraine is a highly individual condition. Each migraineur has a slightly different experience of what migraine is like.

TYPES OF MIGRAINE

Nearly all migraines take one of two forms: *migraine with aura* (which used to be called *classic migraine*) and *migraine without aura* (formerly known as *common migraine*). You may experience only one type, or you may have both.

Migraine Without Aura (common migraine)

Four out of five people with migraine experience migraine without aura. The characteristic feature of a migraine headache is pain on one side of the head, although many people have pain on both sides. The pain may get worse with activity and may seem to throb in time to your heartbeat. Nausea and/or vomiting usually accompany the head pain. For this reason a migraine headache is frequently called a "sick headache." Sometimes the vomiting will be followed by a reduction of your pain. During the attack you may feel the need to get off by yourself in a dark, quiet place and lie down.

People with common migraine may find that they are more easily misdiagnosed and dismissed than people who experience the dramatic aura of a classic migraine.

Elizabeth A. has migraine without aura. For years physicians, family, and friends alike treated her as if she suffered some major defect in character because of her headaches.

"We never get to do anything because you always get a headache" was a sentence she heard over and over from her brothers and sisters while she was growing up. When the physicians she consulted found no brain tumor or other major health problem, the head pain was dismissed as psychological.

If she were recovering from surgery, a broken arm, or even a bad head cold with visible symptoms, Elizabeth would have received a great deal of understanding and help for her problem. But when she had "only" a headache, her nausea, debility, and need for a quiet, dark room were dismissed as histrionics. She knew her headaches were real, but because she lacked the more dramatic signs associated with migraine (such as aura or vomiting) she could not make anyone else accept them as real.

Migraine with Aura (classic migraine)

About one in five people with migraine experiences migraine with aura. Aura is a neurological symptom that occurs before the head pain begins. It may take many forms (see below, "The Forms of Aura"), but usually it is visual in nature. Except for the presence of the aura, all other symptoms of migraine with aura are the same as those of migraine without aura.

Aura is such a startling phenomenon that it often sends someone running straight to the doctor.

Janet M., a woman in her late forties, experienced her first classic migraine during a much-anticipated trip to New York City. She hadn't seen her son in several months, and she was looking forward to staying with him and visiting the museums and art galleries. She felt fine as she boarded the plane. But delays caused by the weather meant she didn't have dinner at the usual time. Instead she ate the typical airplane snack fare: honey-roasted peanuts and diet soda.

By the time the plane landed, Janet noticed that she was having difficulty focusing her eyes. Then a pattern of wavy lines—the aura—filled her visual field for ten minutes. When she arrived at her son's apartment forty-five minutes later, she had full-blown, throbbing head pain.

Although she had experienced headaches all her life, she never had discussed them with her doctor. This one, with its dramatic aura, sent her straight to the emergency room for medication and to a neurologist when she returned home.

LESS COMMON VARIANTS OF MIGRAINE

The following types of migraine are extremely uncommon. Most are variants of migraine with aura. Taken together they account for less than 2 percent of all migraine attacks.

Basilar Migraine occurs primarily in children and adolescents. A form of migraine with aura, its name is derived from the portion of the brain (the base of the brain or the brain stem) that is believed to be involved in the symptoms. The syndrome usually begins with vision problems in both eyes, sometimes progressing to temporary blindness. Vertigo, ringing in the ears, slurred speech, confusion, weakness in the arms and legs, numbness of the tongue and lips, and loss of consciousness may also occur. These symptoms may last up to forty-five minutes and are usually followed by a severe, throbbing headache at the base of the skull. Occasionally some of the symptoms of basilar migraine may outlast the headache, and in rare cases may become permanent. This condition is referred to as migraine-related stroke. (See Chapter 20, "Uncommon Complications of Migraine.")

Hemiplegic Migraine, another rare variant of migraine with aura, occurs mostly in children. In this syndrome paralysis or altered sensation on one side of the body may accompany the aura or the headache. The paralysis may or may not occur on the same side as the head pain. The child may also have problems speaking. The paralysis usually passes quickly, but may sometimes outlast the headache by several days. In rare cases there may be permanent damage. (See Chapter 20.)

Ophthalmoplegic Migraine most commonly occurs in children. Usually the attack begins with a one-sided headache, followed by double vision. The double vision may last three or four days, and sometimes longer.

Ocular Migraine (also called *retinal migraine*) is a type of migraine in which blindness or blurred vision occurs in one eye. Headache on the same side of the head may precede, follow, or accompany the visual symptoms. The visual disturbance usually lasts minutes, but occasionally lasts for several hours. In rare cases the eye is left permanently blind after one or more attacks. Because the symptoms of ocular migraine mimic those of other eye problems, the diagnosis is made only after excluding other possible causes.

Migraine Aura Without Headache, also called *migraine equivalent,* is a broad term that covers several types of migraine. People who experience migraine equivalents essentially have the aura of a migraine without the subsequent head pain. The symptoms of aura are as varied as for any classic migraine. They may include stomach pain (see below), sudden mood change, dizziness, blurred vision, unexpected tiredness and fatigue, food cravings, nausea, or loss of appetite. Some researchers have observed that migraine equivalent often begins after middle age. Others report that these symptoms may appear in children who later develop classic migraine.

Abdominal Migraine, sometimes considered a form of migraine equivalent, is a migraine variant in which all the traditional symptoms of migraine with or without aura appear, but the severe pain occurs in the abdomen instead of the head. Not all researchers accept this type of migraine as a valid entity. Those who do, believe it occurs almost exclusively in children.

Ice Pick Headache is a fragment of migraine characterized by one or more quick stabs of piercing head pain. The pains occur intermittently in various parts of the head. They may last only seconds or continue for several minutes. Ice pick headaches usually occur between more traditional migraine attacks.

THE CHARACTERISTICS OF A
MIGRAINE ATTACK

"When I get that tired feeling around my eyes and can't stand to be in the sunlight, I know I'm in trouble."

"About a half hour before I get a migraine, I get extremely tired and find myself fighting an almost uncontrollable irritation with whoever is nearby—my husband, my kids, my best friend, even the clerk in the grocery store."

Every person with migraine has his or her own "typical migraine," a unique pattern of experiences that occurs before, during, and after an attack. Even within the same person, however, each migraine attack may differ from the typical pattern, and the pattern itself tends to change over time.

Nonetheless, there are strong similarities from attack to attack and from person to person in the *shape* of a migraine attack. In nearly all people a migraine attack is like a bell-shaped curve. There is a period during which activity builds, a much longer time during which the headache is at full intensity, followed by a gradual return to normalcy. Headache specialists usually talk about three phases of a migraine attack; *preheadache, headache,* and *postheadache.* If the person has migraine with aura, the aura typically occurs during the end of the preheadache period.

Phase I: *Preheadache* (also called the *prodrome*) may begin hours to days before the headache begins. During preheadache you may experience mood changes, irritability, fluid retention, increased thirst, or frequent urination.

You also may have food cravings, especially for carbohydrates, candy, or chocolate. Sometimes you will have gastrointestinal symptoms, such as abdominal bloating, stomach rumbling, or constipation. Energy levels vary: some people feel suddenly lethargic, while others are bursting with energy.

- *Aura,* if it occurs, typically begins twenty to sixty minutes before the headache phase. It develops gradually over five to ten minutes, and usually lasts about ten to twenty-five minutes before fading. The headache begins within an hour of the aura's disappearance.

Aura sometimes persists into the headache phase, although it rarely lasts more than an hour. If it does remain longer, it may require special attention from your doctor as a possible precursor of migraine-related stroke. (See Chapter 20.)

The Forms of Aura

Most people who experience aura have visual manifestations, but aura may also include changes in your sense perceptions, movement, speech, or mental functioning. The most common forms of aura include:

- *Visual*
  - A bright shape that spreads across the visual field and appears to block vision, partly or totally, in one eye; it can be seen with eyes open or closed
  - Flashes of light and color
  - Wavy lines
  - Geometric patterns
  - Blurred vision
  - Partial loss of sight
- *Sensory*
  - Numbness or tingling of the face or upper extremity on the same side
  - A sense that limbs are distorted in shape or size or that one foot or hand is larger than the other (sometimes called the "Alice in Wonderland" phenomenon)
  - Odor "hallucinations" (such as floral scents, cooking gas, burning wood chips)
- *Motor*
  - Partial paralysis
  - Weakness or heaviness in the limbs on one side of the body

- *Language*
  - Difficulty finding words
  - Problems understanding spoken or written language
- *Cognitive*
  - Confusion
  - Disorientation
  - Transient global amnesia (similar to the amnesia that follows a concussion)

Phase II: *Headache* is the period during which migraine's most debilitating manifestations—head pain, nausea, and vomiting—occur. Headache may begin at any time, and it is not uncommon to be awakened from sleep with a headache.

The headache stage may last anywhere from four to seventy-two hours. In the uncommon cases where it lasts more than seventy-two hours without improvement, it indicates a serious problem called *status migrainosus,* requiring immediate medical attention. (See Chapter 20.)

Whole-Body Manifestations During the Headache Phase

The altered functioning of the central nervous system leading to migraine may also result in a wide variety of noticeable changes in the body. These can include many striking changes in functioning or behavior:

- *Digestive system*
  - Nausea and/or vomiting
  - Intolerance of food odors
  - Loss of appetite
  - Diarrhea or constipation
- *Skin*
  - Pallor
  - Cold, clammy extremities
  - Facial swelling (edema)
  - Goose bumps

- Bloodshot eye
- "Black eye"
- Facial sweating
- *Fluid Disturbances*
  - Water retention (before and during the attack)
  - Frequent urination (after the attack)
- *Respiratory*
  - Frequent yawning (especially before the attack)
  - Sighing and hyperventilation
  - Nasal congestion and/or runny nose
- *Sensory*
  - Sensitivity to light and noise
  - Intolerance of being touched
  - Heightened sensitivity to odors
- *Mental/Personality*
  - Irritability
  - Depression or anxiety
  - Nervousness
  - Difficulty concentrating

Other, less noticeable manifestations of migraine may also occur, such as changes in the blood chemistry, blood pressure, blood-vessel dilation, temperature regulation, or heart rhythms.

Almost always the changes that take place during a migraine attack are temporary and disappear completely between attacks. In rare cases, however, the aura or the headache and vomiting may be prolonged. One such complication is called *status migrainosus,* mentioned above. Another, called *migraine-related stroke,* is a visual, sensory, or other aura that persists into and beyond the head-pain phase. These uncommon complications always require prompt attention from a doctor. (For more information, see Chapter 20.)

Phase III: *Postheadache* (also called the *postdrome*) is the twenty-four-hour period following the headache. Many people experience fatigue or depression during the postdrome. Others have an opposite experience, reporting feelings of euphoria or intense well-being. Other commonly reported postheadache effects include poor concentration, reduced physical activity, and frequent yawning.

In many people the three phases of the migraine syndrome tend to blend into one another. But becoming more aware of the typical pattern is important. Sometimes an attack can be halted during the preheadache phase by taking quick action in response to early warning signs. (See Chapter 12.)

CYCLICAL PATTERNS OF MIGRAINE

If you have migraine, you may notice that your attacks tend to come in a particular recurring pattern. If you study the pattern, you may find that it corresponds to some triggering factor you encounter on a regular basis.

Three of the most common cyclical patterns are *menstrual migraine, weekend migraine,* and *"letdown" migraine.*

- *Menstrual migraine* is a pattern in which women have monthly attacks at a specific point in their menstrual cycle, usually just before or during their periods or at the midcycle during ovulation. Normal hormonal activity is the probable trigger. For more information, see Chapter 17, "Menstrual Migraine."
- *Weekend migraine* is exactly what it says—migraine attacks that occur regularly on weekends. In many cases the trigger is changing your sleep or eating patterns.
- *"Letdown" migraine* is a phenomenon nearly every migraineur has experienced. You are faced with some major task—a report at work, spring cleaning, giving a dinner party, a family gathering, business travel. You marshal all your energy to succeed, and especially to avoid getting a headache in the process. You perform beautifully—and then just when it's all over and you relax, the headache hits.

The triggers for a letdown headache may be a combination of factors, among them relaxation after stress and fatigue from overexertion.

A recent study suggests that seasonal cycles may also affect the number and frequency of headaches. In this study of patients admitted to a university hospital for treatment of migraine, women were found to be more likely to be admitted during the spring than at any other time. Another study found that time-of-day patterns may also be present. Migraineurs in the study were most likely to have a migraine attack between 6:00 A.M. and 10:00 A.M., and least likely to have one from 8:00 P.M. to 4:00 A.M. Interestingly, heart attacks and other blood-vessel problems show the same time pattern.

CHAPTER 6

Migraine Triggers

Mark K. is an active, healthy man in his early thirties who had never had so much as a tension headache in his life. One spring, however, during a busy season at work, Mark began experiencing a peculiar phenomenon: after a few hours of "feeling weird" he would begin to see a bright, pulsing, strobing light. He could see the light even with his eyes closed, and it stayed in his sight for up to an hour before fading away.

Mark consulted his family doctor, who sent him to a neurologist. After a battery of tests the neurologist told Mark he was experiencing an unusual form of migraine called aura without migraine.

Armed with a migraine diary and the **doctor**'s explanation of how certain factors can trigger **migraine**, Mark hunted for his possible triggers. First he thought the culprit was job stress. Later he discovered something more specific: the sleep disturbances and the enormous quantities of coffee he consumed whenever he worked late.

If you are like most migraineurs, you instinctively recognize that certain things you do or don't do seem to bring on at least some of your migraine attacks. These actions (or omissions) are called *migraine triggers*.

It is critical for you to understand the role that triggers can play in migraine. Learning about your migraine triggers will become an important part in the process of gaining more control over your headaches. (See Chapter 10, "Your Part in the Treatment Process.")

AN ACTIVATOR, NOT A CAUSE

Imagine, for a moment, that your best friend has rigged a pail of water over your doorway as a practical joke. When you open the door, you activate the mechanism, and the water comes pouring down on you.

This imagined scene illustrates precisely the role that triggers play in the chain of events that lead to a migraine. As we have stressed repeatedly, migraine is a physical illness that begins with a physical predisposition (see Chapter 4). This physical predisposition is like the rigged-up pail of water: it is the *cause* of migraine. A migraine trigger merely *activates* that existing physical potential. If you didn't have the potential for migraine, you wouldn't get one no matter what you did to "provoke" it. No pail of water, no mechanism—no shower.

Why is this distinction so important? First of all, you must understand that the trigger does not "make" the migraine. In biological terms the pail of water is already present. Your body may well have been in the process of making the migraine. In all likelihood you would have gotten it eventually. The trigger simply set the process in motion or hastened it along.

It's also important to realize that you are not "guilty" of your headache. If you fell victim to your friend's practical joke, no one would accuse you of *causing* your own drenching, even though it was your hand on the door handle that activated the mechanism. Living with migraine is difficult enough without blaming yourself if you get a headache. A headache is not a sign that you failed to avoid a trigger. The headache might have come anyway eventually, no matter what you did.

You certainly can take steps on your own behalf by learning about triggers and avoiding the obvious ones that bother you. You cannot, however, undo your biological predisposition. This fact explains why some people can avoid all the known triggers and still get debilitating migraines, while others get no headaches, or manageable ones, by avoiding a single triggering factor, such as sleep disturbance or exposure to cigarette smoke.

A SENSITIVITY—NOT AN ALLERGY

Another common misconception about migraine triggers is that they are substances you're allergic to. People frequently make that assumption about dietary triggers. The biological mechanisms of allergy and migraine, however, are very different.

An allergic reaction is a biological process in which your body's immune system (the system that attacks dangerous invaders like bacteria and chemical toxins) is activated in response to your eating, drinking, touching, or breathing any substance to which your body has a strong reaction. The immune-system response leads to the typical symptoms of the allergic response: red eyes, runny or stuffy nose, skin welts, wheezing, and breathing difficulties.

Migraine triggers do not work by stimulating the immune system. So on a biochemical level it's inaccurate to think of yourself as "allergic" to a migraine trigger. It is much more accurate to say that a migraine trigger is a substance to which your nervous system has become sensitized.

Keep in mind, too, that being sensitized to a trigger does not mean it will provoke a migraine every time. The process isn't that mechanical. If your migraines are triggered by red wine, for example, you may not get a headache after drinking one glass at a quiet dinner with friends. But drink that glass during a stressful cocktail party under fluorescent light, and the headache may descend swiftly afterward.

POTENTIAL MIGRAINE TRIGGERS

Triggers can include almost anything in your lifestyle or environment, including foods or beverages, chemicals, sunlight, and hormones.

Even though a predisposition to migraine may be inherited (see Chapter 4), susceptibility to a specific trigger probably is not. Even within a family, individual triggers vary. You may get a headache when a weather front moves in; another member of your family may be affected by cheese, chocolate, and perfumes.

Responses to triggering substances tend to occur within minutes or hours of exposure. For this reason one of the best ways to identify triggers is to keep a headache diary. (See Chapter 10, "Your Part in the Treatment Process.")

Dietary Triggers

Somewhere between 8 and 25 percent of people who experience migraine can point to some particular food or group of foods that may trigger attacks. For a small percentage diet is their only known migraine trigger. Although triggering foods are as individual as the people having the migraines, there are some foods that many migraineurs report as troublesome.

Alcoholic beverages may be the most common dietary trigger. Red wine and beer are among the most likely alcoholic beverages to cause problems. The culprit isn't just the alcohol; another trigger can be found in the *congeners,* the substances that give each alcoholic beverage its particular color, flavor, and aroma.

Tyramine, a chemical found in such foods as aged cheeses, Chianti wine, pickled herring, dried smoked fish, sour cream, yogurt, and yeast extracts, affects several key mechanisms known to be involved with migraine.

Chocolate is another common dietary trigger—an intriguing fact, since many migraineurs report craving chocolate during the preheadache phase of a migraine attack.

Food additives also are often reported as migraine triggers, but it is not clear whether they really precipitate migraine or cause other headaches that share some of migraine's features.

An almost unavoidable additive is the flavor enhancer *monosodium glutamate (MSG).* Many people think of it as being used in Chinese food, but they don't think of it as being used in pepperoni. In fact, MSG is used in virtually all processed foods. It is used in quick and easy microwavable frozen dinners, in canned and dry soups, in prepared tomato and barbecue sauces, in salad dressings and weight-loss powders.

Avoiding MSG, if it seems to trigger your headaches, means cultivating the art of reading ingredient labels. The problem is that a label won't always list MSG as a separate ingredient. It can appear also as any of the following ingredients:

- Hydrolyzed vegetable protein
- Hydrolyzed plant protein
- Natural flavor or flavoring
- Kombu extract

The food additive *sodium nitrite,* another frequently cited headache trigger, is a little easier to avoid. It is found most commonly in hot dogs and luncheon meats.

Many people have reported a swift and severe headache in response to *aspartame* (NutraSweet, Equal), an artificial sweetener that contains the chemical phenylalanine. Some research has suggested that aspartame may decrease central serotonin levels, thus affecting what some believe to be the chief mechanism involved in the creation of a migraine. (See Chapter 4.)

Excessive caffeine is another common headache trigger, though these headaches may only resemble migraine. Caffeine in excess is toxic, and it also can create rebound headaches by increasing the body's expectation for the drug. When the level of caffeine in blood drops, the symptoms of withdrawal, including headache, may set in.

But it's wrong to think of caffeine as all bad. In some cases a strong cup of coffee at the start of a migraine attack may abort the headache or lessen its intensity. Caffeine is a component of many headache medications, including both prescription drugs and nonprescription combinations such as Anacin and Extra Strength Anacin (aspirin plus caffeine) and Extra Strength Excedrin (acetaminophen plus caffeine). Caffeine is used in combinations because it promotes rapid and complete absorption of other drugs. It also is a mild cerebral stimulant that raises the levels of certain neurochemicals, helps sharpen thinking, and reverses the sense of dullness that often accompanies migraine.

Many other foods, such as *dairy products, onions, beans, nuts, fatty foods and citrus fruits,* have been reported to cause headache. The mechanism by which these foods trigger headache is not yet known, nor is it clear whether the headaches that follow exposure to them truly are migraines or just migraine look-alikes.

Environmental Factors

Many migraineurs report that they are extremely sensitive to certain features of their environment. The mechanisms by which these factors trigger migraine are not well understood, but the experience of migraineurs suggests that these sensitivities are powerful triggers.

Light is a problem frequently cited by migraineurs. Bright sunlight can trigger migraine in some people. Flickering lights, the one-after-another popping of camera flashes, or fluorescent overhead lighting can bring on an attack in others.

Strong odors are another common trigger. These odors may include perfumes, fumes from industrial complexes, secondhand cigarette smoke, or air pollution.

Some people with migraine seem to be extremely sensitive to *changes in weather conditions.* Low-pressure weather fronts moving into an area are often cited as particularly troublesome.

Nearly all migraineurs report some problems with *travel.* Airplane travel, for example, exposes a person with migraine to multiple triggers: high altitude, dry air, motion, and noise. Travel by car or train is equally problematic, since many migraineurs experience motion sickness.

The triggering effects of light and motion may be combined when migraineurs look at *complex visual patterns* that seem to move, such as checks or wavy lines. Such patterns can be powerful migraine triggers for some people.

Lifestyle Factors

A common myth about migraine is that it can be caused by factors in the way a person with migraine lives. The implication, of course, is that if people with migraine would just learn to live right, migraine would cease to be a problem for them.

Lifestyle factors do not cause the biological illness of migraine, but they often play a role as triggers of migraine attacks.

Stress, for example, is a potent trigger for many migraineurs. Some researchers have suggested that stress lowers the physiological threshold for a migraine attack by increasing the amount of the hormone adrenaline present in the bloodstream.

Learning to manage stress, if it happens to be one of your triggers, is an important component of managing your migraines. If stress is one of your triggers, it does not mean that you have a weak character, any more than having chocolate as a trigger means you have bad dietary habits. It is important not to chastise yourself for "creating your own migraine" by allowing yourself to be under stress. Stress is as ubiquitous as chocolate—and sometimes equally unavoidable!

A type of stress reaction familiar to many migraineurs is the "letdown" migraine. (See Chapter 5.) In this case it is the letdown period after a stressful situation that tends to trigger the migraine. Stress is not the only lifestyle factor implicated as a potential migraine trigger. *Disturbed sleep patterns,* whether too little or too much sleep or midday napping, commonly set off migraine attacks. Alterations in the brain's blood flow and in the levels of certain brain chemicals during sleep may be ultimately responsible for these migraines. Dreaming, too, may play some as yet unknown role in the process of making a migraine.

Other lifestyle factors that migraineurs frequently cite as problems are *fatigue, skipping meals,* or *eating at irregular or unaccustomed intervals.* Eating a lot of *junk food* also may be a trigger for some people.

Among the most important—and too often overlooked—lifestyle triggers is *smoking.* Migraineurs who smoke risk triggering their headaches, and they also may have less success when using many standard migraine treatments.

Medications

A number of medications, particularly ones that have a dilating effect on the vascular (blood vessel) system, may trigger migraine in susceptible people.

Among the known medication triggers is the drug *nitroglycerine,* used to treat heart disease; *certain drugs for high blood pressure,* such as reserpine and hydralazine; *certain diuretics* (drugs that reduce excess fluid); and *certain antiasthma medications,* such as aminophylline. *Birth-control pills* and *estrogen* also may trigger migraine in some women.

The *too-frequent use of pain medication,* both over-the-counter and prescription drugs, or *overuse of ergotamine* to treat migraine can also result in more frequent migraines. Overuse of these drugs triggers withdrawal headache, which the migraine patient then tries to treat by increasing the dose of the medication. Eventually these rebound headaches become daily events, leaving the patient in far worse straits than ever. Hospitalization is sometimes necessary to break the vicious cycle safely. (See Chapter 21, "Medication Overuse and Rebound Headaches.")

Physical Factors

Head trauma—even a relatively minor injury—can sometimes trigger a migraine attack. Even people with no previous history of migraine may begin having recurrent migraines after a head injury. The injury may activate an existing predisposition to migraine. (For more information on migraine and head injury, see Chapter 4, especially the section, "Is Migraine Inherited?") Certain invasive medical tests, such as angiography or myelography, may occasionally have the same result.

Sudden or intense exertion, which every migraineur knows can make a migraine headache worse, also can trigger migraines in some people. Sexual orgasm, for example, whether occurring during intercourse or other forms of sexual activity, may trigger a headache.

Some sports, such as tennis, racquetball, jogging, or jumping rope, seem to be particularly likely to trigger attacks. The reason may have something to do with the quick motions and eye movements these activities require.

Migraines brought on by exertion should be reported to your doctor, particularly if they are very severe. They may simply be garden-variety migraines, but sometimes they signal other disorders of the blood vessels in the head.

Hormonal Factors

Nearly any biological event that causes a change in the production or balance of hormones is a potential trigger for a woman whose migraines are linked to her menstrual cycle (see Chapter 17, "Menstrual Migraine"). These events include menarche (the beginning of menstrual periods), monthly menstruation, menopause, pregnancy and delivery, or taking hormones in the form of birth-control pills or for estrogen replacement therapy after menopause or a hysterectomy.

Paradoxically, nearly all the factors that act as hormonal triggers for some women may signal a reprieve from migraine for others. Pregnancy, in particular, seems to temporarily inhibit migraine for many women.

KEEPING TRACK OF YOUR MIGRAINE TRIGGERS

Check off any factors that seem to bring on your migraines. Then use this list to help you fill out your headache diary. (See Chapter 10, "Your Part in the Treatment Process.")

Dietary Factors

Alcoholic beverages	[ ]

Foods containing tyramine
aged cheeses	[ ]
Chianti wine	[ ]
pickled herring	[ ]
dried smoked fish	[ ]
sour cream	[ ]
yogurt	[ ]
yeast extracts	[ ]

Chocolate	[ ]
Citrus fruits	[ ]
Dairy products	[ ]
Onions	[ ]
Nuts	[ ]
Beans	[ ]
Caffeine (excess, withdrawal)	[ ]
Fatty foods	[ ]

Food additives
Nitrites (e.g., in hot dogs, luncheon meats)	[ ]
MSG	[ ]
Aspartame artificial sweetener (NutraSweet, Equal)	[ ]

Environmental Factors

Bright light	[ ]
Flickering light sources	[ ]
Fluorescent lighting	[ ]
Perfumes	[ ]
Strong odors	[ ]

Fumes from industrial complexes [ ]
Air pollution [ ]
Secondhand cigarette smoke [ ]
Motion [ ]
Travel [ ]
Complex visual patterns (e.g., checks, zigzag lines) [ ]
Weather changes [ ]

Lifestyle Factors

Stress [ ]
Disrupted sleep patterns [ ]
"Letdown" [ ]
Fatigue [ ]
Irregular eating habits [ ]
Cigarette smoking [ ]

Medications

Blood vessel dilating drugs (e.g., nitroglycerin) [ ]
Drugs for high blood pressure (e.g., hydralazine, reserpine) [ ]
Diuretics [ ]
Antiasthma medications (e.g., aminophylline) [ ]
Too-frequent use of analgesics, ergotamine [ ]

Physical Factors

Head trauma [ ]
Invasive medical tests (adverse effect) [ ]
Exertion (e.g., sports, sexual orgasm) [ ]
Disorders of the neck [ ]

Hormonal Factors

Menarche [ ]
Menstruation [ ]
Menopause [ ]
Pregnancy [ ]
Delivery [ ]
Birth-control pills [ ]
Estrogen replacement therapy [ ]

CHAPTER 7

Migraine
and Other Types
of Headache

As someone who is predisposed to have headaches, you may find that you experience several other types of headache in addition to migraine. You may also find that some other type of headache is mentioned by your doctor as a possible alternative diagnosis to migraine. Or if your headaches are especially severe, you may wonder whether your doctor hasn't "missed something" and assigned you the wrong diagnosis.

Understanding the range of headache types other than migraine may help you gain greater confidence that migraine really is the correct diagnosis for your condition. And if you do experience several types of headache, it may help you get a better handle on which symptoms go with which type of headache so you can give better information to your doctor.

MAJOR CLASSIFICATIONS OF HEADACHE

Despite the controversies among researchers about whether headache is one disease or many (see Chapter 4), physicians who treat headaches take a practical approach. They typically classify headache on the basis of symptoms. These clinical classifications and qualifying symptoms were regularized in 1988 by the International Headache Society (IHS), an organization of headache researchers and clinicians from around the world.

The IHS defined four major diagnostic categories for primary headaches—that is, headaches that do not result from other diseases. In addition to migraine with aura and migraine without aura, the other two major types are **tension-type headaches** and **cluster headaches.**

Tension-Type Headaches

Suzanne S., a self-employed consultant who works out of her home, had just spent a long weekend at the beach relaxing. Arriving home after a four-hour, nonstop drive, she went into her office and began listening to her phone messages. The first was from her accountant—a cryptic message about a call he had received from the IRS. The second was from an important client, asking her to attend a vital meeting in two hours.

After a hasty shower and a change of clothes, she made the meeting with just minutes to spare. As the client's new financial manager droned on for an hour in an overly warm room, she fretted about the call from the IRS. Soon she began to feel a tight, viselike pressure around her head.

Suzanne's headache was a typical tension-type headache. Although many of these headaches have no obvious trigger, hers was probably brought on by a combination of emotional, physical, and environmental stresses. Tension-type headaches, which account for about 90 percent of all headaches, are often described as dull, tight, squeezing pain around the back of the neck, the scalp, and the forehead. The pain is typically mild to moderate, less intense than a migraine headache but troublesome nonetheless.

Exactly how and why these types of headaches arise is not known. Some researchers believe they are not really distinct from migraine—just a milder form. Others see them as a completely different disorder, possibly developing from scalp-muscle tension.

From the headache patient's point of view tension-type headaches differ from migraine in several important ways. For one thing, they can be much shorter than migraine or much longer: they typically last anywhere from thirty minutes to seven days. They also may be more frequent: while migraineurs usually have one to three migraine attacks per month, chronic tension-type headaches can occur daily or every other day.

Tension-type headaches feel different from migraine: they press or tighten rather than throb, and they often are present in both sides of the head. They also differ in that they are not usually as debilitating as migraine: there is no nausea or vomiting, and physical activity doesn't aggravate the pain.

Tension-type headaches are annoying and can interfere with your daily enjoyment of life, especially if they occur frequently. In many cases, however, they can be controlled by mild pain relievers such as aspirin or acetaminophen and relaxation techniques.

Cluster Headache

Bob R., a man in his mid-thirties, was awakened from sleep at four A.M. by a searing pain just above his left eye. He knew immediately what he was in for, because a similar pain had awakened him nearly every night for the past week.

His eye began to tear, and his nose felt runny; these, however, would prove to be little more than annoyances when compared to the head pain. The headache was excruciating, like a hot poker in the eye. He got up and paced around the bedroom, grinding his fist into his eye. His wife found him minutes later, sitting in a chair in the den and repeatedly banging his forehead against a textbook.

Bob's experience was a classic example of a cluster attack. As the name implies, the headaches typically occur in clusters. An attack usually lasts from fifteen minutes to three hours and may occur one or more times a day, every day, in clusters that last for weeks or months. The headaches generally happen at about the same time each day, often beginning during sleep.

Cluster headache is distinctly different from migraine. Like migraine the pain of a cluster headache is localized on one side of the head, but the focal point of a cluster headache is very specific: usually in or around the eye or in the temple. The eye on the pain side may become red and teary; the eyelid may droop and the pupil may contract. There may also be nasal congestion or discharge and facial sweating.

Cluster headaches are excruciatingly painful, even more so than severe migraine. The pain of a cluster headache is usually not throbbing, but is often described as boring, drill-like or "like a hot poker in the eye." The pain is so intense that people have been known to injure themselves by banging their heads against walls or other objects in an attempt to gain relief.

Whereas migraine affects more women, cluster headache occurs most often in men. They are usually heavy smokers.

HEADACHE TYPES IN COMBINATION

If you have migraines, you may experience tension-type headaches between migraine attacks. About 10 percent of all tension-type-headache sufferers also experience migraine. Some physicians call this a *mixed headache syndrome.*

It is less common, but not unknown, for a person with migraine also to experience cluster headaches.

The presence of more than one type of headache sometimes

complicates the process of diagnosing the headache disorder. Treatment for all three types of headaches may overlap, since many of the same drugs and nondrug therapies are helpful for all three.

CHRONIC DAILY HEADACHE

Sybil E., a woman of thirty-one, had had migraine without aura since puberty. For years she had been self-treating each attack with several doses of aspirin, which never succeeded in bringing much relief.

Her attacks gradually increased in frequency from once a month to once a week, and she sought a physician's help. The physician gave her a prescription painkiller with a narcotic, and she began taking these as well as her customary doses of aspirin.

Instead of improving, however, the headaches became more frequent and less responsive to the medication. Over the course of several months she took more and more pain pills, but her headaches gradually became daily events.

Chronic daily headaches like the ones that Sybil E. developed usually evolve from migraine. In about half the cases they occur in people who take certain over-the-counter or prescription headache painkillers too often, causing a rebound effect. These patients usually experience quick improvement when they are withdrawn from their medications under a doctor's care. (See Chapter 21, "Medication Overuse and Rebound Headaches.")

LESS COMMON TYPES OF HEADACHE

Migraine, cluster, and tension-type headaches account for as much as 95 percent of all headaches. But there are other headache varieties as well. Although they are far less common, accounting for no more than 5 percent of all headaches, they are important for you to know about. Sometimes they provide an early warning of tumors, allergies, infection, disorders of the blood vessels in the head, or exposure to toxic substances.

Even if you are taking medicine for migraine, be sure to see a doctor if you begin getting headaches like any of those listed here, or if your headaches change and start to feel different from those you've had in the past.

Headaches That Result from Organic Diseases

Head injury headache (also called posttraumatic headache) may occur after even a minor injury. The headache can recur for months or even years after the original injury. Although usually benign, it sometimes signals a subdural hematoma, or blood clot pressing on the brain. If you develop head pain after a head injury, be sure to have the headache evaluated by your doctor, especially if the pain gets progressively worse.

Sinus headache is a common self-diagnosis whenever pain occurs over the sinus cavities. True sinus headache, however, is relatively uncommon and accompanies acute sinus inflammation. Many people who are certain they have chronic sinus headaches actually are experiencing migraine.

Hypertension headache is not associated with common high blood pressure. It is a rare condition that is the result of sudden rise in blood pressure in the 250/100 range.

Aneurysm headache is a sudden, severe headache. It is worse than any previous headache and is often accompanied by stiffness in the neck. An aneurysm is the ballooning of a blood vessel. Its slow leak or rupture causes a hemorrhage into the head. An aneurysm headache may be accompanied by mental confusion and loss of consciousness or signs of a stroke. This type of headache requires immediate medical attention.

Meningitis headache produces intense head and neck pain and stiffness of the neck. Caused by an inflammation of the membranes around the brain and spinal cord, it results from bacterial or viral infection. These headaches are usually accompanied by fever, malaise, and severe debility.

Brain tumor headache usually begins with intermittent head pain that gradually becomes more frequent and severe. Many times people with brain tumors do not initially experience headaches. Instead, they experience slurred speech; motor, sensory, or visual symptoms; personality changes, or seizures.

Temporal arteritis headache begins after the age of 55. The headache is due to inflammation of the temporal artery or other scalp artery. It may be accompanied by aches in the body or extremities and by visual symptoms. If untreated, it may lead to blindness or a stroke.

Headaches from Other Causes

Chronic Paroxysmal Hemicrania is a rare headache, usually seen in women. Its symptoms are similar to that of cluster headache: episodes of severe pain around the eye, accompanied by eyelid swelling and drooping, tearing, or nasal discharge. The attacks last one to two minutes and occur as many as a dozen or more times a day.

Exertion headaches occur during exercise, coughing, sneezing, or sexual activity. They are typically brief, throbbing headaches, and they usually are not serious. However, it is important to discuss them with your doctor. Sometimes these headaches are symptoms of a tumor, aneurysm, or blood-vessel malformation.

TMJ syndrome headache is a dull, nagging pain, aggravated by chewing, in the area of the jaw joint (temporomandibular joint, or TMJ). The pain of TMJ syndrome is thought to be caused by misalignment of this joint. The usual symptom is tenderness over the joint in front of the ear. Many physicians believe TMJ syndrome, like sinus headache, is a common misdiagnosis for headaches caused by other problems.

Carbon monoxide headaches are triggered by exposure to carbon monoxide and produce throbbing pain, dizziness, weakness, and nausea. Toxic levels of carbon monoxide can be emitted from a defective furnace or from a defective auto exhaust system. Carbon monoxide builds up in the bloodstream over time, so even short exposures in a car can be dangerous if repeated day after day.

Eyestrain headaches usually occur in the forehead after reading in poor light or working at a computer too many hours. They may signal the need for reading glasses or for taking more breaks during the workday.

Hunger headaches usually are generalized pain in the head. They occur just before mealtime or when meals are skipped.

Hangover headaches occur the morning after drinking too much alcohol. They are probably due to the effect of alcohol withdrawal.

Caffeine-withdrawal headache occurs when a daily coffee-drinker skips the morning brew. The pain may be localized or generalized and may be accompanied by fatigue or irritability.

Ice cream headache occurs briefly in the forehead and temples. It is caused by eating ice cream or cold foods too rapidly. Scientists are not sure why these headaches occur.

MSG headache produces migrainelike throbbing pain in the temples and forehead and tightness and pressure in the face. MSG is monosodium glutamate, a flavor enhancer used in Chinese food and many processed food products.

Don't Ignore These Warning Signs!

Even if you have had headaches for many years, see your physician or go to an emergency room *immediately* if you experience any of the following symptoms:

- Sudden, severe head pain
- Head pain accompanied by fever
- Progressively worsening headache, especially following an injury to the head

- Head pain accompanied by mental confusion, seizures, mood swings, or other neurological symptoms
- Headache that begins after exertion, straining, coughing, or sexual activity
- First headache problem that begins after the age of fifty-five
- Headache that occurs daily or interferes with the quality of life

Any of these symptoms may turn out to be harmless, but sometimes they signal a serious underlying condition that requires immediate attention.

PART TWO

Treatment
for
Migraine

CHAPTER 8

The Migraineur's Bill of Rights

Two out of three migraineurs are not currently seeing a physician. Nearly one in five have *never* consulted a physician.

A patient survey reported at the International Headache Congress in 1991 noted that of 136 chronic headache patients, only 30 percent were fully satisfied with their treatment; 45 percent said their medicine didn't work, and one out of three felt their physicians were poorly informed about their condition.

If you are like many people who get migraine headaches, you may never have seen a physician to get help for your headaches. Maybe you dismissed your pain by saying it was "just a headache" —not something that should send you to the doctor.

If you have tried to get help, the odds are you gave up after the first try—either because the doctor didn't take you seriously, or because the medicine didn't seem to work. And if your headaches are so bad that you just *couldn't* give up, you probably have seen a lot of doctors by now—between five and eight, on average.

If you went to the doctor with a broken arm, you'd feel you had a *right* to be treated. You would be shocked and angry if the doctor seemed disinterested or uninformed. You would expect a certain level of care—and you would probably get it. And you would expect your health-insurance carrier to reimburse you appropriately for necessary medical treatment.

It is time migraineurs recognized that they have the *right* to receive treatment, just like a person with a broken arm. Granted, it may be difficult to stand up for that right. Traditionally, we accept what the doctor says, with no questions asked. But that attitude can cost you a lot of unnecessary suffering—because there are treatments available that are likely to work for you, and growing numbers of doctors who will listen to you.

For this reason we feel it is important to start our discussion of treatment with a "Migraineur's Bill of Rights." Read it over, think about it, discuss it with your doctor and family—and take it to your heart. You deserve to receive help!

For some of the ideas in this bill of rights, we are indebted to Herbert G. Markley, M.D., a Worcester, Massachusetts, headache specialist, and to other physician members of the American Council for Headache Education who frequently make presentations on the subject.

THE MIGRAINEUR'S BILL OF RIGHTS

1. I have a right to be taken seriously by my physician when I go for treatment of my headaches.
2. I have a right to a complete and thorough medical examination, including a medical history and complete neurological evaluation.
3. I have a right to appropriate diagnostic testing, including neurodiagnostics, CT scans and MRI scans, if necessary,

when my headaches are first evaluated *and* when the headache pattern or severity changes.

4. I have the right to be referred to a specialist—for example, a neurologist, a headache specialist, or a headache clinic—if my headaches do not respond to my primary physician's treatment, or if my primary physician feels a specialist's care is needed.

5. I have the right to receive specific headache therapy, if needed, instead of nonprescription drugs, narcotics, or combination analgesics that may increase the problem.

6. I have the right to ask for a comprehensive, written treatment plan that will tell me exactly how to use my preventive medications and nondrug preventives and that will provide complete instructions on what to do when a headache occurs.

7. I have the right to return for additional help whenever my treatment plan seems to be inadequate to control my headaches.

8. I have the right to be treated courteously and responsibly in emergency rooms, if a severe headache fails to respond to my usual treatment plan.

9. I have the right to expect my insurance company to recognize migraine as a legitimate illness, and to persist in appealing any denied claims for legitimate medical care that would be covered for other illnesses.

10. I have the right to expect those around me—family, friends, co-workers, and others who come in contact with me—to make an effort to understand my illness and to cooperate with me in my efforts to live a full, rich life.

CHAPTER 9

Finding the Right Help

"The average person who calls me has been to about fifteen doctors."

—Ruthe Ragsdale, cofounder of
headache support groups in
Colorado and Florida

Having a chronic illness like migraine means that you will inevitably spend a lot of time and money on medical care. To achieve the best possible outcome when you seek treatment for migraine, the most important step in the whole process takes place right at the very beginning: finding the right help.

"The right help" is a physician who is caring, knowledgeable, and compatible with your personal style. He or she may be a headache specialist, a headache researcher, or your family doctor. The key element is not necessarily the doctor's area of specialization, but whether you feel you can build a long-term, satisfying relationship of trust and honesty—a relationship in which your need for relief from migraine is understood and honored. You must feel comfortable that the physician is interested in keeping up with the scientific study of migraine and in undertaking the long, collaborative treatment process with you.

The quality of the patient-physician relationship is critically important, because treating migraine is not a "cookbook" process. There's no one right answer for everyone. In many instances you and your physician will be exploring the options together, trying and eliminating many medications before finding the one that works best with the fewest side effects. The medications may stop working for you after a time, necessitating another round of trial and error. During this process you must be able to talk frankly with your doctor about what you did or didn't do that may have affected the success of the treatment, without worrying that you will be judged or chided if you encounter a trigger or fail to follow the treatment plan to the letter.

THE TREATMENT PARTNERSHIP

For migraine patients the best model for relationship building is the relationship that diabetics, asthmatics, and other patients with chronic, episodic illnesses develop with their doctors. This relationship is called a *treatment partnership.* The word *partnership* implies that both parties have an important role to play in keeping the patient well.

A treatment partnership has three important characteristics:

- **Long-term Commitment.** Doctor and patient both realize that they will have a long-term relationship, working together to keep episodes of illness to a minimum and to treat them promptly when they occur.
- **Realistic Goals.** Doctor and patient both realize that no prevention plan can eliminate bouts of illness from time to time. Instead, the goal is gaining the longest possible period

of illness-free living with the maximum quality of life during treatment.

- **Joint Efforts.** Doctor and patient jointly agree on a treatment plan that the patient is willing and able to follow and that balances the benefits of medications and other therapies against the problems caused by their side effects.

How will you know when a doctor is willing to build this kind of relationship with you? You will have to probe for information that will help you evaluate the doctor's commitment to caring for migraine patients.

Considerations About the Doctor

- Is the doctor interested in treating migraine? Is he or she knowledgeable about the latest theories on migraine and the current research on migraine treatment?
- Does the doctor seem willing to listen to your feelings about how well a particular medication works for you? Will he or she change the medication if you find the side effects or the medication schedule unworkable?
- Will the doctor give you a written treatment plan, including an "emergency plan" if none of your regular treatments seems to help?
- Do you feel you can talk honestly to this doctor about your condition, without feeling judged if you get a headache despite treatment?

Because treatment is a partnership, it's not just the doctor you have to evaluate. You also have to examine whether *you* are motivated for the treatment process. To achieve better control of your condition you must be prepared to make a commitment to self-care and to cooperating with your physician.

Considerations About Yourself

- Are you willing to accept the fact that finding the right treatment for your migraines may take time and may involve trying some treatments that don't work?
- Are you ready to accept responsibility for your part in the treatment process? (See Chapter 10.)
- Are you willing to be open-minded about nondrug treatments that will require an investment of time and energy? (See Chapter 15.)
- Can you be open with your physician about your financial situation, so that ways of paying for needed treatment can be explored?

Questions to Help You Choose a Doctor for Migraine Treatment

When you call for an appointment to see a physician about your migraines, tell the receptionist that you have some questions to ask the doctor and that you'd like to make sure there is time in the schedule.

Don't be shy about asking your questions. If the doctor isn't comfortable taking the time to talk to you, that may be a sign you need to look elsewhere for help.

1. **Have you treated many migraine patients?**
   A doctor who often treats migraine is most likely to be familiar with the latest treatment plans.
2. **What do you believe causes migraine?**
   The doctor should be familiar with the latest understanding of migraine as an illness that affects brain chemicals.
3. **In your experience, does treatment work for migraine?**
   Your doctor should view migraine as a highly treatable (though not curable) illness—not as something you may have to just "live with."
4. **If you prescribe something that doesn't work very well**

or that makes me feel bad even if it gets rid of my headache, what would you do?

The doctor should be willing to try other medications and nondrug treatments to see if something else gives you an outcome that seems better to you.

5. **Will you give me a written treatment plan to follow?**
Any doctor should say yes to this request. The treatment plan should explain how and when to use all your medications and should include specific instructions for what to do when your usual medications fail to help.

6. **Do you ever refer your migraine patients for nondrug treatments like biofeedback?**
A doctor who is knowledgeable about migraine should say yes or be willing to consider this option.

7. **What did you do when one of your migraine patients didn't get any relief from the usual treatments?**
The doctor should have some sort of escalation plan—such as referring you to a neurologist or headache specialist.

8. **Is there someone in your office who can help me with financial issues related to treatment?**
An affirmative answer is important to help relieve you of the stress of the financial aspects of migraine treatment.

LEVELS OF CARE FOR MIGRAINE HEADACHES

When you look for medical care for your headaches, it is a good idea to be familiar with the various levels of care available to you. Although most people start with their own physicians, you do not have to stop there if you don't find relief. Many other avenues are open to you to find the right help for your headaches.

Who Treats Migraine Patients?

- Primary-Care Physician
- Medical Specialist
- Neurologist
- Headache Specialist
- Headache Treatment Program
- Chronic Pain Treatment Program

Primary-Care Physician

The primary-care physician is the physician that most people see first for routine care or treatment of illness. In health maintenance organizations and many other forms of health insurance coverage, the primary-care doctor is a "gatekeeper," who decides when you need to see other specialists.

Usually the primary-care physician is a general practitioner, family practitioner, or internal-medicine specialist. Some women use their gynecologists as their primary-care doctors.

Advantages in migraine treatment:	■ Knows your whole medical picture ■ May treat other family members ■ Presumes a long-term treatment relationship
Disadvantages:	■ May not have sufficient familiarity with current research on migraine and latest treatment protocols ■ If the primary-care physician is the gatekeeper to other specialists, may not consider migraine serious enough to warrant referral
When to seek this level of care:	Unless you are experiencing symptoms that require emergency care (see the "When to Seek Help . . ." box following this section), start here to see whether you can receive the help you need.

When to
bypass this
level of care:
There's no need to stop here if your doctor doesn't give you specific and helpful treatment. Ask for a referral to a neurologist or headache specialist, or go on your own.

Medical Specialists

Some people who experience migraine go to specialists because they are worried about specific symptoms that accompany migraine: for example, if you begin experiencing migraine aura for the first time, you may think you are having eye trouble and consult an ophthalmologist.

You also may be sent to one or more medical specialists when you ask your primary-care physician to give you help with your headaches. Sometimes the consultation can uncover previously unsuspected problems that cause migrainelike headaches or aura.

Specialists that migraine patients often see are endocrinologists, orthopedists, ophthalmologists, gynecologists, rheumatologists, otolaryngologists, allergists, and dentists or oral surgeons. (For more information about the functions of each of these specialists, see Chapter 11, "Diagnosing Migraine.")

Advantages
in migraine
treatment:
▪ These physicians can identify uncommon causes of headache that may mimic migraine.

Disadvantages:
▪ These physicians often spend a lot of time— and money—looking for uncommon causes of your symptoms without first considering the possibility that you are experiencing migraine.

When to seek
this level of
care:
For most migraine patients, specialists need not routinely be consulted to make a diagnosis. Usually you should consult your primary-care physician first before self-referring to these specialists.

When to bypass this level of care: Unless there are specific indicators in your medical history, your family's medical history, your physical examination findings, or your routine medical tests, you usually should not be referred to these specialists for diagnosis of head pain. Ask your doctor to tell you exactly what factors are leading him or her to refer you. If you're not satisfied that there's good reason, ask for a referral to a headache specialist instead. If you decide to accept referral to other specialists, don't undergo expensive tests or procedures without first getting a second opinion, preferably from a headache specialist.

Neurologist

A neurologist specializes in diseases that affect the brain, and hence is highly qualified to diagnose and treat head pain and other migraine symptoms. Primary-care physicians often refer patients with headache to these specialists to confirm the diagnosis of migraine; other times they refer because they suspect that the head pain is not caused by migraine.

Advantages in migraine treatment:
- Because they have specialized knowledge of the brain and its functioning, they can identify the presence of uncommon neurological disorders that cause migrainelike head pain.
- They are likely to be familiar with current theories of migraine and have at least a general familiarity with treatment options.

Disadvantages:
- Not all neurologists are **especially** interested in headache treatment.
- Patients with the more severe forms of migraine usually are referred to neurologists, but their practices may not be equipped to pro-

vide the necessary support, referrals, and follow-up care as you try to establish the best headache regimen for you.

When to seek this level of care: If you have not been able to get relief through the treatments offered by your primary-care physician, or if there are suspicious neurological findings in your history, physical examination, or routine tests, a neurologist is often the logical next step.

When to bypass this level of care: If there are no suspicious neurological findings in your medical history, your family's medical history, your physical examination findings, or your routine medical tests, but you have not yet found relief after trying a number of treatments offered by your primary-care physician, you should try to determine whether there is a headache specialist, clinic, or center in your community and ask for a referral there instead.

Headache Specialist

A headache specialist is a physician—usually a neurologist, but sometimes an internal medicine specialist or other medical specialist—who diagnoses and treats head pain.

Advantages in migraine treatment:
- Likely to have the most detailed knowledge of current treatments for migraine.
- Likely to be efficient and cost effective in diagnosis.

Disadvantages:
- Headache is not a defined medical subspecialty with specific accreditations, so you cannot immediately be certain of the background and credentials of someone who says he or she is a headache specialist. One way of

establishing the person's level of professional interest in headache is to determine whether he or she belongs to organizations such as the American Association for the Study of Headache (AASH), a professional group for physicians and researchers interested in headache. (For more information on AASH, see the "Resources" at the end of this book.)

When to seek this level of care: If you have tried working with your primary-care physician but have not achieved a reduction in the frequency and severity of your headaches, or if you are taking painkillers more than three days a week, a headache specialist may be able to try newer or more aggressive treatments. To find a headache specialist affiliated with AASH in or near your community, contact the American Council for Headache Education (ACHE). (See "Resources.")

Headache Treatment Program

Several dozen specialized headache treatment programs are now in place around the country. These programs usually are headed by a headache specialist, who works with a multidisciplinary team of physicians, nurses, psychologists, and other clinicians whose primary interest is in finding the optimum treatment for each patient's headache condition.

Many of these programs are little more than outpatient clinics that provide evaluation and referral to professionals in the community. Some, however, are substantial, well-thought-out programs with multidisciplinary specialists practicing under one roof. A few of these programs are located in or affiliated with hospitals. The inpatient component of the program provides inpatient care to wean people from ineffective medications, get a patient through a crisis of *status migrainosus* (see Chapter 20), test a variety of possible treatments in a controlled environment, or find the right medication for patients who have other complicating medical conditions such as systemic lupus erythematosus or diabetes.

Advantages in migraine treatment:	• These programs are expressly designed to meet the needs of headache patients and incorporate a variety of support systems for effective follow-up and a sustained treatment relationship.
Disadvantages:	• Since there are no national standards that define what a "headache treatment program" should include, not all programs are comprehensive or include the full range of diagnostic and treatment modalities.
When to use this level of care:	Migraineurs who have not found significant relief from their headaches after working with a primary-care physician, neurologist, or headache specialist should consider a headache treatment program.

Most headache programs accept self-referrals, although they usually prefer you to be referred by your physician. At least one headache treatment center has voluntarily sought and received accreditation by the Council on Accreditation of Rehabilitation Facilities (CARF). CARF is a national body whose accreditation means the program has met strict standards for clinical programs, patient care, treatment outcomes, record-keeping, and financial management. As more headache treatment centers seek and achieve accreditation by a legitimate accrediting agency, this accreditation will help patients feel secure about the quality of care they receive and will encourage uniform standards of care. To find out whether there is a headache treatment program in or near your community, contact ACHE. (See "Resources.")

Chronic Pain Treatment Program

Many communities have hospital-based programs to treat people with chronic pain resulting from illnesses or injuries. Often the people admitted to these programs are taking more pain medication than they should; some may even be physically addicted to their medications.

Some communities also have outpatient pain programs that either supplement the inpatient program or substitute for it, particularly when the pain patient is not addicted to any medications. These programs are often similar to headache treatment programs, although their patients may have many different kinds of pain other than head pain.

Advantages in migraine treatment:

- Chronic pain management programs wean patients from overused pain medicines.
- These programs are often multidisciplinary in nature, looking to a variety of medical and ancillary fields for ways to manage pain without chronic use of pain medication.
- Many of these programs acknowledge the impact on the patient's family and involve the family in the treatment process.

Disadvantages:

- The programs often focus on getting patients off ineffective painkillers and do not have enough time to fully investigate the potential for migraine prevention through carefully chosen preventive agents.

When to use this level of care:

If you do not live near a headache center, and you have headaches nearly every day or are taking painkillers more than three days a week, a chronic pain program may be able to help you deal with rebound headaches (see Chapter 21). Usually you cannot self-refer to these programs; your primary-care physician or headache specialist must admit you. If your doctors aren't enthusiastic about the idea, but you want to investigate whether the program can help you, contact the office of the program's director; he or she will refer you to a doctor who can evaluate your condition and decide whether you might be helped by participating in the program.

When to Seek Help (and from Whom)

IF . . .
- you have been having the same type and number of migraine headaches for many years
- they come less than once a month
- you can successfully manage them with nonprescription painkillers taken at the doses recommended on the label

. . . you probably don't need or want any special treatment for your headaches. **BUT IF YOU HAVE NOT YET DISCUSSED YOUR HEADACHES WITH YOUR PRIMARY-CARE PHYSICIAN, DO SO AT YOUR NEXT VISIT.** Your doctor will probably agree with you that no special care is needed, but you should *never* self-diagnose your headaches.

IF . . .
- you have headaches that come once a month or more
- that make you miss work or school
- that last for more than a day
- that don't go away when you use nonprescription painkillers
- that are accompanied by nausea or vomiting

. . . you can be helped by seeing a doctor knowledgeable about the treatment of migraine. The sooner you seek help, the sooner you can find effective relief. **DO NOT DIAGNOSE YOUR OWN HEADACHES OR SELF-TREAT WITH MORE THAN THE RECOMMENDED DOSES OF NON-PRESCRIPTION PAIN KILLERS.**

IF . . .
- you have sought medical help for your headaches but did not find relief
- you stopped a prescribed medication because you didn't like the side effects
- you find yourself going to the emergency department for a narcotic every time you get a severe headache
- your headaches used to be every once in a while, but now are daily or almost daily
- you take nonprescription medications at higher-than-recommended doses and/or more than four days out of the week

. . . you probably should consult a headache specialist, a headache clinic, or a comprehensive headache treatment center. Do not give up on your medical options. **DO NOT DIAGNOSE YOUR OWN HEADACHES.**

IF . . .
- you are having your *first* headache or your *worst* headache
- you are having any unusual neurological symptoms (such as vision problems, weakness or paralysis in a limb, confusion, slurred speech)
- your headache is accompanied by fever or stiff neck

. . . **SEEK IMMEDIATE MEDICAL CARE AT AN EMERGENCY DEPARTMENT!**

THE ROLE OF THE HOSPITAL EMERGENCY
DEPARTMENT IN MIGRAINE TREATMENT

The hospital emergency department plays a similar role in the treatment of migraine that it does in the treatment of other chronic recurrent illnesses: the place of last resort when your treatment plan fails, and the first place to go if unusual and alarming symptoms appear.

Even if you are following your treatment plan carefully, you may find yourself with a migraine that does not respond to the medication-escalation plan your doctor outlined. This is not your fault—it is one of the mysteries of migraine. Asthma patients, diabetics, and others with chronic illnesses experience similarly inexplicable medication failures from time to time.

Anytime you go to an emergency department or walk-in urgent-care center for treatment of migraine, be sure to follow up with your regular doctor promptly. Your doctor will want to evaluate your treatment plan to look for any possible explanation for its failure and to make sure it still is appropriate for you.

What Emergency Departments Can Do
to Help Migraine Patients

Many migraine patients feel that emergency departments treat them with disrespect and with disregard for the seriousness of their condition. Emergency-room personnel, they say, do not consider severe migraine a true emergency. Instead, they bombard hapless migraineurs with demeaning questions and imply that they are drug abusers seeking a narcotic fix.

"I have a foolproof method for dealing with insensitive emergency-department doctors and nurses," said one woman who has had severe migraine for twenty years. "I throw up on their shoes."

You do have a right to prompt, caring attention in an emergency department. But consider the task of the emergency-department personnel. They must quickly assess the status of many people, some of whom may be experiencing immediately life-threatening medical conditions. They must keep a responsible eye on medications, and that means weeding out drug abusers, notorious in urban emergency departments especially, who can't afford street drugs and come to the emergency department with imaginary pain that can be cured only by a shot of narcotics.

Headache experts, physicians, and headache patients in many communities have begun to work with emergency-department personnel to develop a standard emergency-department protocol for handling migraine patients. Here is one possible form the protocol may take, based on suggestions by a group of researchers who attended a 1990 roundtable on the treatment of intractable migraine:

Emergency Department Migraine Treatment Protocol

1. Immediately place the patient in a quiet, dark room.
2. Take a headache history to find out whether the patient has had similar headaches in the past.
3. Check vital signs and neurological-status indicators.
4. Rule out ominous causes of headache, such as meningitis or subarachnoid hemorrhage.
5. Administer appropriate abortive treatment: DHE, sumatriptan, or the treatment recommended by the patient's personal physician.

One way you can assist the emergency-room personnel is by always carrying with you a copy of your treatment plan, which should include your physician's name, telephone number, and DEA registration number, your diagnosis of migraine, and a record of the medications your doctor prescribes. (See Chapter 12.)

JUDGING "SUCCESS" IN TREATMENT

When you go to the doctor with an ear infection, you know exactly how to judge whether treatment was successful: you wait to see if the infection goes away. With migraine, however, as with asthma or diabetes, the underlying disorder is not going to go away. It can't. It is part of your body's built-in physiological makeup.

One of the most difficult aspects of having a chronic illness is accepting the fact that the illness will recur from time to time—no matter how careful you are and no matter how excellent your medical care. You can avoid every trigger, take your medicine as directed, live a totally stress-free life—but you cannot control all the factors that go into making a migraine deep inside your brain, and you cannot control all the biochemical factors that affect how your medicine works.

Managing your migraines also takes a lot of hard work. Unfortunately, people with chronic illnesses cannot take for granted many of the simple activities of life. Think about diabetics, for example: they have to monitor their diets strictly, check their blood sugar, estimate their insulin needs, and inject themselves several times a day. Or asthmatics: they take powerful medications daily, check their lung capacity frequently with a peak flow meter, and pretreat themselves with special medicines if they might be exposed to potential triggers in the environment.

As a migraineur you're in the same situation. You have to keep alert for migraine triggers that may be in your diet or your environment, monitor the warning signs of an impending headache, and find a way to treat yourself immediately when one begins.

Because migraine medications are powerful drugs that affect your brain chemistry and blood vessels, they also tend to have many possible side effects. These side effects can range from annoying (such as a dry mouth) to troublesome (such as aching muscles or memory problems) to frightening and potentially dangerous (such as muscle spasms or chest pains).

When you go for treatment of migraine, it is up to you to

decide how to balance your need for relief against the inconveniences and side effects of treatment. For this reason treatment "success" for migraine is defined in a highly subjective and fluid way as *attaining the greatest amount of control over the condition with the maximum quality of life during treatment.*

The trade-off between "control over the condition" and "quality of life" is highly personal. If a medication could reduce your headaches from three a month to one a month, but you were groggy until noon each day as a result, would you take that medicine? If you have just one truly awful headache a month, would you be willing to take a preventive agent twice daily? If you know that changes in altitude may trigger your headaches, are you willing to let your family go to the mountains on a ski trip without you?

It will be up to you to decide what trade-offs you are willing to make and to communicate that information to your doctor. That way both of you will be evaluating the success of your treatment from the same perspective.

MIGRAINE TREATMENT AND MONEY

There is no denying that medical care costs money. Medical care for chronic, episodic illnesses like migraine can be very expensive. For example, the most common diagnostic tests used to rule out dangerous causes of migrainelike headaches (see Chapter 11) may cost upward of $1,000. If your headaches are severe and frequent, the mix of medications prescribed for prevention and treatment may cost $100 to $200 a month or more. Newer medications may be even more expensive. For people whose condition seems intractable, a stay in a hospital-based headache unit or chronic-pain unit may cost $2,000 to $8,000 or more.

If you have health insurance, your insurer may pick up some or all of these costs. Sometimes you may have to go through a lengthy process to collect appropriate reimbursement (see Chapter 30). Your doctor can be your ally in this process. Right at the start of your treatment it is very important to talk to the person on your doctor's staff who handles health insurance. That person can help you determine how much coverage you have and what forms and receipts you must submit to speed up the reimbursement process. In addition, your doctor usually must receive preapproval (called *precertification*) before your insurance company will pay for expensive diagnostic tests or for hospitalization.

If you do not have health insurance, or if you are worried that you will have trouble covering the uninsured part of your medical care, it is essential for you to talk this over with your physician and with the financial manager on your physician's staff. Sometimes payment plans can be worked out, or your community may have medical-care credit programs. If you cannot afford to pay for care, you may qualify for financial-aid programs, clinic care, or other help. Some centers around the country do have special charitable programs for people in desperate financial straits who also have desperate headaches. Do not assume that you have to suffer just because you do not have financial resources.

CHAPTER 10

Your Part in the Treatment Process

"When you're trying to get good treatment for migraine, the most important thing is not to give up. Plus, you have to take responsibility to take care of yourself—not just wait for doctors to take care of you. Everybody is different; you are the one who knows you best."

Because the treatment process for migraine is an active partnership between you and your physician, your commitment to the process is just as important as your physician's. And just as the physician has a responsibility to know and use the latest information to devise potentially helpful treatment plans, you have a responsibility to gather and communicate other information crucial to treatment. This information is about you: your habits, your lifestyle, your headache patterns, your pain perception, your ability to follow the treatment regimen and your successes or failures when you do.

As with other chronic illnesses like asthma or diabetes, your ability to communicate effectively about your migraines and to provide the physician with as much clear information as possible can have a tremendous influence on the effectiveness of your treatment regimen.

CREATING YOUR MIGRAINE PROFILE

Going to the doctor can be an anxiety-provoking experience. You wait, fill out forms, take tests, then spend time with the nurse and the doctor answering questions and being examined. In this environment it's easy to forget important facts you want to communicate about your headache history—facts that may be vital in helping your physician understand your condition.

To make sure you communicate everything of importance, prepare a migraine profile to take with you to the doctor. Your migraine profile contains all the pertinent facts about when your headaches started, what they feel like, how you now treat them, and what made you decide to ask for more help. The profile also includes all the questions you'd like to have answered.

To help your physician determine your unique migraine profile, make a copy of the form below, fill it out, and take it with you when you consult your doctor. The filled-out sample profile may help you in determining how to complete the form.

YOUR MIGRAINE PROFILE

Name:

Age at first headache:

Why you are seeking treatment for headache now:

Headache frequency and duration:

Has headache frequency recently changed?

Typical symptoms (location, preceding or accompanying symptoms):

How painful (on a scale of 1 to 4)?

Have headache symptoms recently changed?

Related to menstrual cycle?

Possible triggers (diet, other factors):

Family history of similar headaches?

Current treatment:

Other treatments tried:

Questions to ask:

SAMPLE MIGRAINE PROFILE

Name:	Anne X.
Age at first headache:	14
Why you are seeking treatment for headache now:	Headaches disappeared for a few years, now are back
Headache frequency and duration:	2–3 times a month
Has headache frequency recently changed?	Yes—more frequent
Typical symptoms:	Fatigue, nausea, blurred vision
How painful (on a scale of 1 to 4)?	3 to 4
Have headache symptoms recently changed?	Never had vision problems before
Related to menstrual cycle?	No
Possible triggers (diet, other factors):	Always get a headache after drinking red wine. Frequently get one after eating mushrooms or cheese. Get headaches when I'm in fluorescent lighting.
Family history of similar headaches?	Mother and sister have sick headaches.
Current treatment:	Fiorinal whenever I need it.

Other treatments tried: Aspirin, ibuprofen, Anacin, Tyle-
                                        nol, Tylenol 3
Questions to ask: Is there something I can do about
                                        the nausea? I'm scared to drive
                                        because the blurred vision
                                        comes on so suddenly—what
                                        can I do?

COMMUNICATING CLEARLY ABOUT PAIN

"Having a migraine is nothing like having a headache,"
one longtime migraine patient says flatly. "It's more like
having your head stepped on by a herd of cattle."

Many people with migraine believe that the people around
them confuse the pain of migraine with the pain of so-called tension-type headaches. One way to cut down the frustration of trying to get others to understand how you feel is to make sure you
and those in your life, including your physician, are speaking the
same language. "I have a horrible headache," or "My head is
pounding and feels like it's going to explode," may not mean the
same to any two people—especially to someone unfamiliar with
the pain of migraine. And even in a group of migraineurs it is
good to have some way of communicating your unique experience
of pain.

Many migraineurs and physicians suggest setting up your own
pain rating system using a scale of 1 to 4. Define what *your* head
pain feels like at each stage. Write down the definitions. Then give
them to your family and to friends who know you have migraine.
Take them with you to your doctor. That way, when you say you're
between a Level 2 and 3, the doctor will know exactly what you
mean and will know what interventions to take.

MY HEADACHE PAIN RATING SYSTEM

Level 1:

Level 2:

Level 3:

Level 4:

SAMPLE HEADACHE PAIN RATING SYSTEM

Level 1:   Bad head pain, but I can still function as if everything is okay. I'm usually feeling depressed at this point.

Level 2:   Moderately bad head pain with some stomach symptoms (mild nausea, vomiting, diarrhea). I still can function okay in routine activities such as typing, driving, or preparing dinner, but don't ask me to do anything more. I'm starting to lose my grip, and my thinking is getting muddled.

Level 3:   Awful head pain with pronounced stomach distress. Light, sounds, and odors make my head hurt worse. I can't think clearly, and I don't think I'm going to be good for anything much longer. I feel so bad, I could cry.

Level 4:   Excruciating head pain, vomiting, impaired reasoning, and sensitivity to light, sounds, and odors. I'm incapable of functioning at all now. I'm in agony. All I want is to be lying down in a dark, silent room.

KEEPING A HEADACHE DIARY

Once you have begun working with your doctor to treat your headaches, it is wise to keep a headache diary. It can speed diagnosis by your doctor, help you keep track of treatments, and help you and your physician monitor the effects of treatment. It can also help you decide whether a treatment is failing or whether some special circumstances (for example, forgetting to take your preventive medication for a few days, or taking an airplane trip, or losing sleep during a stressful period at work) might be making the medication temporarily less effective.

The headache diary is a record of the circumstances before, during, and after a migraine attack. Obviously you may not feel like recording everything that is happening to you while it is happening. But if you can't, you should try to fill out the diary as soon as you can after you feel better, so that you won't lose any important details. Include as much information as you can so that when you take it to the doctor, he or she can see what has helped and what hasn't.

Use the form below to help you create your own headache diary. Fill it out as soon as you are able when you experience a migraine attack. The sample on the following page can help you understand how to record your migraine information.

MIGRAINE DIARY

Date Migraine Attack began: Time:

Duration of attack (from preheadache through headache to end of postheadache phase):

Preheadache symptoms:

Level of pain during headache (1 to 4):

Any stomach distress
(nausea, vomiting, diarrhea):

Sensitivities during headache:

Medications taken within 48 hours of start of attack:

Name	**Time**	**Dosage**	**Results**

Triggers encountered within 48 hours of start of attack:

   Foods

   Sleep

Weather

Other

Any unusual postheadache experiences/sensations?

Other notes:

_____

_____

SAMPLE MIGRAINE DIARY ENTRY

Date Migraine Attack began: May 6   Time: 2:45 P.M.

Duration of attack (from preheadache through headache to end of
postheadache phase):   Approximately 6 hours

Preheadache symptoms: Tiredness in my eyes

Level of pain during headache (1 to 4): Arrived as Level 2, eventually
became Level 3; skipped Level 1 altogether

Any stomach distress   Nausea only
(nausea, vomiting, diarrhea):

Sensitivities during headache: Light and noise were very painful

Medications taken within 48 hours of start of attack:

Name	Time	Dosage	Results
Tylenol	2:45	2 extra-strength	No help
Anacin	4:15	2	Some help, but pain returned
Anaprox DS	6:00; 6:30	2 each time	First ones helped some, second dose knocked it (and me) out

Possible triggers encountered within 48 hours of start of attack:

Food
Chinese food for lunch (MSG?)

Sleep
7 $\frac{1}{2}$ hours (normal)

Weather
Sunny and mild

Other
Played ball at lunchtime, delayed my usual meal by an hour; no other unusual activities

Any unusual postheadache experiences/sensations?
Felt sluggish and unable to think clearly when I woke up.

Other notes:
I wish I had taken the Anaprox first, but I was afraid it would irritate my stomach. Need to ask doctor if I can take a drug for the nausea with Anaprox.

KEEPING A WATCH FOR MIGRAINE TRIGGERS

An important part of preventing migraines or lessening their frequency is knowing and avoiding your migraine triggers. Triggers are highly individual, and only you can discover them by closely observing the circumstances immediately preceding the onset of your headaches.

To become familiar with your possible triggers, take inventory by filling out the chart that appears in Chapter 6. Then use your headache diary to keep track of triggers that you may have encountered before each migraine attack.

CHAPTER 11

Diagnosing Migraine

"I've been to everything short of a witch doctor."

Many migraineurs tell stories of going from doctor to doctor seeking an explanation for their head pain. The truth, however, is that migraine is not a difficult disorder for a knowledgeable physician to diagnose, even though there is no one test, no one physical finding, that definitively says "migraine."

Your doctor should be able to determine whether your headaches are caused by migraine disorder or some other cause by:

- Taking a good headache history.
- Giving a simple physical exam.
- Ordering a few diagnostic tests to rule out other possible causes of migrainelike headaches.

THE MIGRAINE WORKUP

When you first go to your physician to seek help for your head-aches, you should be prepared to spend at least thirty to forty-five minutes with the physician and his or her staff. During this time they will be looking for information and physical findings that *rule out* other causes of your headaches and that *point to* migraine as the cause.

Reason for current visit

Your physician will want to know why you are coming in now to seek help for your headaches. For example, you may have begun experiencing headaches more frequently, or you may have had unusually severe or prolonged headaches. Or you may have begun having aura, or noticed a change in the aura. You may have begun having physical symptoms that are unusual for you, such as weakness in a limb or mental confusion.

Thorough headache history

Your physician will ask when you began having headaches, what triggers them, what they feel like, how long they last, who else in your family gets them, and other information. If you have created your headache profile (see Chapter 10), you should give your physician a copy for his or her files.

Physical exam

During a physical examination your physician usually will check the following:

- **Vital signs** (heart, lungs, blood pressure, temperature)
- **Eyes,** to make sure pupils respond normally and to look for unusual swelling or redness

- **Ears, nose, mouth, and throat,** to look for signs of infection or sinus problems
- **Neck,** to see that it has normal flexibility
- **Head,** to check for unusual contours or sore spots
- **General observation of strength and sensation in face, arms, and legs,** to check that both sides of your body are responding normally
- **Reflexes,** to test general functioning of your central nervous system

COMMON DIAGNOSTIC PROCEDURES

If you have never had a headache workup before, if you have changed doctors, or if you have experienced changes in the type or frequency of your headaches, your physician may want to run a number of diagnostic tests. The tests listed here are not unusual, and it should not alarm or surprise you if you're asked to take them.

Lab tests

Your physician usually will order a few simple blood tests to look for changes in blood chemistry that may suggest underlying disorders needing further investigation. There currently is no blood or other lab test that can "prove" you have migraine; these tests simply rule out other possible causes for your symptoms.

Diagnostic imaging

To rule out any hidden organic cause of your headaches, such as tumors or blood-vessel abnormalities, your physician may send you to have diagnostic imaging of your brain. Like blood tests, these images cannot prove you have migraine; they simply confirm that you don't have any other illness or problem that could be causing your head pain.

If you have obvious migrainelike symptoms, a history of similar headaches, no ominous warning signs, and a family tree full of migraineurs, your physician may tell you the diagnostic imaging is not necessary. Treatment will then proceed on the assumption that you have migraine. If you don't respond to treatment as expected, or if the headaches worsen despite treatment, you may be sent for diagnostic imaging at a later time.

If you do have diagnostic imaging, your physician will generally order a *CT scan* or an *MRI*.

CT scan.   CT, or computerized tomography (sometimes called a CAT scan), is an X-ray technique. First, you may be injected with a contrast dye. Then you will be placed in the tunnel of the CT scanner, a sophisticated X-ray machine that will take pictures of thin cross-sections of your brain at a number of angles. The procedure usually takes about thirty minutes (although the latest generation of CT scanners works considerably faster). CT scanning is painless, except for the minor discomfort of the dye injection.

MRI scan.   MRI, or magnetic resonance imaging, does not use X rays or X-ray dyes and is completely painless and harmless. For an MRI scan you are placed inside the MRI machine's large cylindrical tunnel, which contains a strong magnet. The magnet temporarily affects the nuclei of the hydrogen atoms in your body, making these nuclei line up in a pattern that matches the magnetic field. The energy released when the magnet is off and the atoms realign will be picked up by a receiver in the MRI machine, which records all this activity, feeding the information to a computer. The computer is programmed to use this information to construct a picture of the tissue being studied. The picture is projected on a TV screen, and it can also be saved on film for additional study. An MRI scan usually takes between thirty and sixty minutes. Some people report feeling claustrophobic while in the MRI tunnel, but the current generation of MRI scanners has many features to help make the experience more pleasant.

OTHER DIAGNOSTIC TESTS

Occasionally you may be asked to take other diagnostic tests, especially if the physician has reason to suspect that your headaches are not caused by migraine. These tests include:

Angiogram (or **Arteriogram**). An X-ray study of blood vessels in the brain. A contrast dye is injected to make the vessels visible on the X-ray film. This test also shows the arteries carrying blood to the brain.

Spinal tap. Insertion of a needle into the spinal canal to withdraw spinal fluid for study. Some people report discomfort during or after this procedure, but it is usually minor.

Electroencephalogram (EEG). A recording of the brain's electrical impulses to search for unusual activity that indicates disease of or injury to the brain. The EEG tracings are recorded by attaching tiny electrodes to the scalp. These electrodes are harmless and cause no pain or discomfort.

PET scan. Positron-emission tomography, or PET scanning, can gather information about the brain's structure, blood flow, and activity levels. For a PET scan you are first injected with a compound that contains a radioactive isotope. These isotopes attach to a variety of chemicals, such as glucose, that the brain uses for fueling its activities. The PET scanner measures certain particles, called *positrons,* that are emitted as the radioisotope decays. The more positrons detected from a part of the brain, the more activity is taking place there. Aside from the minor discomfort of the injection, PET scans are entirely painless.

Keep in mind that these tests are *not* routine tests for migraine. If your physician asks you to have them, ask for a detailed explanation of why they are indicated. If you are not comfortable with the explanation, you may want to seek a second opinion from a headache specialist.

REFERRAL TO OTHER SPECIALISTS

When you ask your primary-care physician for help with your headaches, you may be referred to one or more medical specialists in a wide variety of disciplines. Sometimes your physician makes the referral because he or she has reason to suspect a specific physical problem that requires specialized treatment. Occasionally a consultation with a medical specialist will uncover previously unsuspected problems that cause migrainelike headaches or aura.

Among the specialists you may consult or be asked to consult with are the following:

Orthopedist—to determine whether problems with bones or muscles, especially in the neck or spine, may be causing or contributing to head pain

Ophthalmologist—to look for eye problems that may be causing headache or aura

Endocrinologist—to look for uncommon biochemical causes of migrainelike symptoms involving the body's hormone-secreting glands, such as thyroid disease

Allergist—to look for allergies that may be causing reactions such as watery eyes, sneezing, wheezing, or breathing problems and that may complicate the process of diagnosing your headaches

Otolaryngologist—to look for ear, nose, throat, or sinus problems that occasionally are the cause of chronic headaches

Gynecologist—to evaluate the possibility that organic disease of the reproductive system may account for hormone-related headaches

Rheumatologist—to look for diseases of the connective tissue, such as systemic lupus erythematosus, which may be accompanied by migrainelike symptoms

Dentists and oral surgeons—to look for dental or jaw problems that may cause migrainelike pain or contribute to triggering migraine

For most migraine patients these specialists need not be consulted routinely to make a diagnosis or to provide effective care for your migraines. Many times such referrals cause medical bills to mount while providing little or no relief.

Be especially cautious if you are tempted to seek out one of these specialists on your own, without your doctor's referral. Many migraine patients go from specialist to specialist looking for "the answer" to their headaches. But if you have migraine, there is no simple answer. Yours is a chronic condition that probably will improve with proper treatment but cannot be cured.

Even if it is your doctor making the referral to one of these specialists, you should still be cautious. Don't automatically assume that "doctor knows best." Ask for a detailed explanation. Was there some finding in your exam or tests that leads your doctor to suspect a specific problem? If you are not convinced of the necessity of the referral, you may want to self-refer to a neurologist, headache specialist, or headache clinic. (See Chapter 9.)

ACCEPTING THE DIAGNOSIS

Some people find it hard to believe that the disconcerting aura, excruciating head pain, intense stomach distress, and other symptoms they experience are caused by migraine. It is very common for migraineurs to harbor a secret fear that they have a brain tumor or some other ominous cause of head pain. Sometimes this secret fear will prevent a migraineur from sticking faithfully to a treatment regimen.

If you have these fears, discuss them with your doctor. Unlike migraine, most other illnesses that cause severe headache have specific physical indications that show up in the examination, blood tests, scans, or other diagnostic procedures. Ask your doctor to go over your test results with you in detail until you feel reassured.

CHAPTER 12

Medications
for Migraine:
General Information

In a recent Roper survey of American health attitudes, more than one third of the people surveyed said they would rather "just live with" a headache until it passes than take medication.

In another survey of more than 20,000 U.S. households, 17.6 percent of females and 5.7 percent of males reported having migraine headaches. Of these, only 41.1 percent of females and 28.3 percent of males said they used prescription drugs to control pain.

Only a small percentage of migraineurs who can be helped by medications actually are receiving them. The pattern of avoiding medicines cuts across economic and social classes—so lack of money to buy medicines is not the major cause of the problem. The most common reasons for this pattern of undertreatment are fear of medication, misunderstandings about how to use medications, and lack of information about medications.

Migraine medications are powerful drugs. When they are administered under the care of a knowledgeable physician, they can bring significant relief to most people who experience migraine. The more you know about migraine medications, the less fearful you will be of trying them and the more prepared you will be for the sometimes complicated process of finding the ones that work for you.

In this chapter you will find out general information about the types of migraine medications, how they're selected, how to take them, and how to avoid some of the common problems and pitfalls. In Chapters 13 and 14 you'll find detailed information on the drugs themselves: what they are, how they work, and the common side effects they cause. At the end of Chapter 14 you'll also find case studies of people who have been significantly helped by migraine medications.

TYPES OF MEDICATION FOR MIGRAINE

Migraine medications fall into two general categories: *medications for the acute attack* and *medications that help prevent attacks.*

- **Acute medications** (also called interventional medications, rescue medications, or abortive medications) are used when a headache is in progress, to stop the head pain, stomach distress and other acute symptoms. Common acute agents are discussed in Chapter 13.
- **Preventive medications** are taken on a regular schedule, whether headache is present or not, to alter the mechanism underlying a migraine and thereby reduce the likelihood of headaches developing. Common preventive agents are discussed in Chapter 14.

If your headaches are relatively infrequent, occurring less than once a month, your doctor probably will not recommend preventive medications. Instead he or she will try to find acute medications that work well to stop your headaches. If you have severe headaches that come two or more times a month, however, your doctor may suggest starting you on a preventive drug with acute medications as backup.

There's no formula for selecting the specific migraine medication that will work for you. When you have an infection, your doctor determines what kind of germ has caused the problem, then selects an antibiotic known to kill that type of germ. With migraine the process is more complicated. Some medications work well for some people and not at all in others. The selection process is largely trial and error, starting with the medications that have the fewest side effects and the smallest risk of addiction or other complications.

THE MIGRAINE TREATMENT PLAN

For chronic episodic illnesses like asthma, diabetes, or migraine, patients often are given a written treatment plan that lists what they are to do at different stages in an episode of illness.

Having the plan in writing can be very helpful. For one thing, you can use it to help your spouse, family members, or others around you understand what to do when your headaches get bad. For another thing, you can take it with you to an urgent-care center or emergency room so the doctors there will know what medicines you're already taking. Your physician also may give you a special letter to accompany the plan, for use during a migraine crisis that results in a visit to an emergency room. The letter may contain the specific emergency-treatment procedures and medications your physician prefers for your care and may help you avoid misunderstandings when you are traveling or using an unfamiliar emergency room.

Here's what a treatment plan might look like:

MIGRAINE TREATMENT PLAN FOR SUSAN T.

Name: Susan T.
             123 Anywhere Drive
             Hometown, VA 22212
Physician: Myron Doctor, M.D.
             (212) 555-1234
             DEA Registration #100000022000

Diagnosis: Migraine without aura

Preventive Treatment: Drug A—1 tablet daily at 8 A.M.

Acute Treatment: Drug B—2 tablets at onset of headache, with one tablet of Drug C if nausea and vomiting are present. Lie down in a dark, quiet room for 45 minutes. Apply hot or cold compresses, if desired.

   If headache improves but does not disappear completely within 45 minutes, take another tablet of Drug B. Continue resting quietly and applying hot or cold compresses.

   If headache worsens during the 45-minute period, self-inject one dose of Drug D. Continue resting quietly and applying hot or cold compresses.

Emergency Treatment: If headache is unusually painful or is accompanied by unusual symptoms, or if none of these measures helps, go to the nearest hospital emergency department and have them contact me at (212) 555-1234. Give the emergency-department personnel this treatment plan and my emergency-care letter containing further instructions.

AN IMPORTANT CONSIDERATION: FOLLOWING THE MEDICATION SCHEDULE

A recent study found that approximately half of those who experienced recurrent headaches did not stick to their prescribed medication schedules. The same study found that as many as two thirds of the migraineurs did not make the best use of the medicines prescribed to stop a headache in progress.

People who do not follow the directions for taking their medications may be losing much of the relief they would otherwise get with these medications. For example, the average patient has about a 40 percent reduction in headache activity when using ergotamine tablets, a common migraine medication (see Chapter 13). But in a recent study patients who were given additional education on how to use ergotamine properly saw a considerably greater reduction in their headache activity.

When medications are developed and approved for use, they are put through rigorous tests to determine the correct dosages and times of administration. In addition headache specialists continually try out new ways of administering medications. The medication schedule your doctor recommends is based on these research findings.

It is important to follow your doctor's directions for when and how to take your medications. *A medication for migraine cannot work unless it is properly used.* If you don't understand the directions, or if you have questions about when and how to take your medicine, call your doctor and ask for clarification. You can also ask the pharmacist who fills your prescription to give you practical advice on how to take the medication, such as whether the medication can be taken with food and what to do if you miss a dose.

If the side effects of a medication are so unpleasant that you can't follow the directions, go back to your doctor and report the problem. *If you are taking preventive medications daily, it is also important to follow your doctor's instructions for stopping them.* Some of these medications, especially those that affect blood pressure, can cause serious problems if they are not withdrawn carefully.

Many people take too little medication because they are *afraid* it will be bad for them—not because of any specific side effects. One woman who had excruciating migraines with prolonged aura threw out her prescription for Inderal, a common preventive medication (see Chapter 14), because a cousin who was taking the drug for high blood pressure had been warned not to discontinue the drug suddenly. Instead of asking her doctor or pharmacist to explain this warning, she decided the warning meant the drug was too dangerous for her to start taking it "just for headaches."

TOO MUCH OF A GOOD DRUG CAN BE BAD

"With each migraine headache I became so afraid of having another that I found myself taking painkillers more and more often," said Sarah T., a woman in her thirties who had experienced migraine since adolescence. "I was so focused on getting rid of each headache that I hardly realized they were coming more and more frequently, until they were an almost daily event."

Severe migraines are so painful and so disruptive that many people start taking their painkilling medicine when there is the slightest hint that a "number 4" headache may develop. The problem is, these medications are not meant to be used in this way. The results of using medications too frequently are as bad as using them too infrequently.

If the dose your doctor prescribed isn't doing the job, you may need a different medicine—not a bigger dose. If a medicine that has worked for you in the past seems to be losing its effectiveness, you may need a change in medication, not more of the same.

This principle also holds for nonprescription medicines. After a certain dose you won't get more pain relief by taking additional doses of aspirin or acetaminophen or ibuprofen tablets. You'll just increase the chances of getting negative side effects and of getting rebound headaches when the drug levels in your blood fall. Overuse of your acute or "rescue" medicines also may interfere with the benefits of your preventive medicines. (For more information, see Chapter 21, "Medication Overuse and Rebound Headaches.")

MEDICATION INTERACTIONS

Prescription and nonprescription medicines you take for conditions other than migraine may change the way your body responds to your migraine medications. They may make your migraine medications less effective, or make it harder for your body to clear the medications from your system. Sometimes they may even boost the action of your migraine medications in ways that are dangerous for your system.

If you go to more than one doctor, it is very important that each doctor is aware of all the medications you take—even over-the-counter antacids or vitamins. Some people recommend the "brown bag" technique: scoop up all the medicines you take, put them in a small paper bag, and bring them along when you visit your doctor. Another safety check is in using the same pharmacy to fill all your prescriptions. Many pharmacies now use computer profiles of each patient to keep track of medications and to alert the pharmacist when interactions are possible.

Another possible source of interactions is allergy treatment. If you are planning to take allergy injections, be sure to tell your allergist about the medications you take for your migraines. Certain combinations of medications and allergy shots may cause unexpected reactions.

MIGRAINE MEDICATIONS DURING PREGNANCY

Many medications for migraine should not be taken during pregnancy. Aspirin and nonsteroidal antiinflammatory drugs (NSAIDs —including over-the-counter NSAIDs such as Motrin IB, Advil, Nuprin, and other forms of ibuprofen) are not advisable for pregnant women. Meperidine (Demerol), codeine, and acetaminophen can be used in pregnancy for acute headaches, but Demerol and codeine are addictive, and overuse of acetaminophen can lead to rebound headaches.

If you are pregnant or plan to become pregnant within a few months, talk to your physician about altering or discontinuing your medications. One possible alternative is using biofeedback, a nondrug therapy that is safe for use during pregnancy. (See Chapter 15.)

If you are lucky, you may not have to worry about your headaches at all during pregnancy. In many women, especially women whose migraines come in sync with their menstrual periods, pregnancy brings temporary relief from migraines.

DO MIGRAINE MEDICATIONS LOSE THEIR EFFECTIVENESS OVER TIME?

A migraine medication may become less effective for you after you have used it for a while. With some drugs the body develops *tolerance.* In other words, your system gets used to having a certain baseline of the medication in your bloodstream, and you need more of the medication to achieve headache relief. The problem is, you can't keep increasing the dosage of most medicines. The higher the dose you take, the greater the likelihood of unwanted side effects, such as rebound headaches, addiction, kidney and liver overload, and other physical problems.

In other cases the body appears to develop *resistance* to a drug's effects. That is, the drug no longer has much effect on your headaches at any dose. It is not known how or why resistance develops. To avoid resistance and tolerance many physicians will change your preventive medications after you have been using them for six months.

Developing tolerance or resistance can be frustrating, especially when you have gotten used to being able to knock your headaches out quickly with a certain dose of a certain drug. Tolerance and resistance are an unpredictable part of what happens when you treat a chronic illness like migraine. Don't be discouraged. Just go back to your doctor and try again.

CHAPTER 13

Medications for Migraine: Acute Treatment and Pain Relief

In the acute phase of a migraine attack, when all the migraine symptoms are present in full force, migraine treatment has three specific aims:

- to relieve head pain;
- to relieve gastrointestinal symptoms (nausea, vomiting, diarrhea);
- to help the patient sleep.

More than one medication may be needed to achieve these goals. Sometimes, the patient may also use nondrug therapies, in conjunction with medication, to make the attack less painful. (See Chapter 15.)

In the discussions of drugs in this chapter and in Chapter 14, each drug will be identified by its chemical or generic name, with common U.S. trade names given in parentheses afterward. These lists of trade names are illustrative, not exhaustive; many drugs, for example, are sold under different names outside the U.S., and new forms of a drug may be sold under different names. If you do not find the trade name of your migraine medication listed here, ask your doctor or pharmacist to tell you the drug's generic or chemical name.

RELIEF FROM STOMACH DISTRESS

Medications for Gastrointestinal Symptoms of Acute Migraine

- Gastrointestinal stimulants
  - metoclopramide (Reglan)
  - domperidone (Motilium)—not yet available in the U.S.
- Nonstimulants
  - prochlorperazine (Compazine)
  - hydroxyzine (Vistaril, Atarax)
  - promethazine (Phenergan)
  - trimethobenzamide (Tigan)
  - chlorpromazine (Thorazine)
  - thiethylperazine (Torecan)
  - dimenhydrinate (Dramamine)

Studies have shown that as many as 95 percent of migraine patients experience gastrointestinal symptoms such as nausea, vomiting, and diarrhea. Many researchers believe the same disturbance of serotonin that causes the head pain also causes the migraineur's acute stomach distress.

To quell these gastrointestinal symptoms physicians may prescribe *antiemetic* drugs. These usually are taken fifteen to thirty minutes before any pain medicine or ergotamine.

The antiemetic drug most commonly used in the U.S. for migraineurs is metoclopramide (Reglan). Metoclopramide is very effective at reducing nausea and vomiting.   It also seems to improve the absorption of certain oral drugs, including aspirin and other painkillers, and therefore may make some of these drugs faster-acting and more effective.

Metoclopramide halts nausea and vomiting by affecting the brain's receptors for the neurochemical dopamine.   Like other drugs that affect the dopamine receptors, it often causes fatigue or sedation and may occasionally cause troublesome (although almost always temporary) side effects, known as *extrapyramidal effects,* in a small number of people. These include various movement disturbances, such as restlessness, involuntary grimaces or limb movements, and symptoms similar to those of parkinsonism.

A newer drug, called domperidone, is not yet available in the U.S. Domperidone works like metoclopramide but is less likely to cause extrapyramidal effects.

The major tranquilizer prochlorperazine (Compazine) acts as an antinauseant and also helps relieve pain. Sometimes it may head off the migraine completely if given early enough. Like metoclopramide it (and other major tranquilizers) may cause fatigue, sedation, and extrapyramidal symptoms. Recent studies suggest that Domperidone may even have some possible use as a migraine preventive agent.

Hydroxyzine (Vistaril, Atarax) and promethazine (Phenergan) are antihistamines which act as mild antinauseants and may also provide some pain relief.

Other drugs that are used to treat nausea in migraine are the motion-sickness drug dimenhydrinate (Dramamine), the antiemetic trimethobenzamide (Tigan), and the major tranquilizers chlorpromazine (Thorazine) and thiethylperazine (Torecan).

If the initial dose of an antinausea drug does not completely resolve the symptoms, it usually is repeated in four to six hours.

RELIEF FROM PAIN

Types of Pain Relievers for Acute Migraine

- Simple Analgesics
- Combination Analgesics
- Specific Antimigraine Drugs
- Major Tranquilizers
- Narcotics
- Corticosteroids
- Minor Tranquilizers

The head pain reported by people who experience migraine usually ranges from moderate to severe to excruciating. The chief goal of acute therapies is to stop the pain as quickly and completely as possible while causing the fewest side effects.

The difficulty is that the course of any particular headache is unpredictable: what worked well last month may not work at all today. As in chronic conditions such as asthma, the physician often will prescribe an "escalation regimen." That is, the migraineur will be instructed to start treatment with one drug, then escalate to another if the first drug proves ineffective or only partly effective within a certain period of time.

Most migraineurs start with a simple analgesic, then progress to a combination drug or an ergot derivative. If none of these treatments work, the patient usually is instructed to take sumatriptan, dihydroergotamine (DHE), or a narcotic.

For migraine patients nearly all pain-relief therapies have one major drawback: they are not as effective if taken long after the headache pain sets in. The only exceptions to this rule are sumatriptan and DHE, both of which are often highly effective even if taken when the headache pain is at full force.

The role of caffeine in treating acute migraine pain deserves a special mention here because many people are confused about caffeine. Caffeine is an important ingredient in many medications used to control headaches. It has several actions that might explain its potential value:

- Caffeine acts as a brain stimulant and affects certain brain chemicals in a way similar to other drugs that help headache. Recent evidence suggests that caffeine may have an analgesiclike effect.
- Caffeine enhances the stomach's ability to absorb medication.
- Caffeine, through its stimulant effect, may help reverse the sedated or cloudy feeling that frequently accompanies migraine.

For most people the caffeine present in antimigraine drugs will pose no problem at all. In fact, some people report that they get better results from painkillers that don't contain caffeine (e.g., aspirin or acetaminophen) if they take them with a cup of coffee or a cola drink.

Caffeine can become problematic for migraine patients, however, when it is used excessively. More than 500 mg of caffeine a day (about the amount in three strong cups of coffee) for several days can lead to more migraine headaches through the rebound effect or caffeine toxicity. In addition, if you habitually ingest caffeine during the day, you may experience caffeine withdrawal at night and be awakened by a migraine.

Simple Analgesics for Migraine

- Aspirin (Bufferin, Ecotrin, Empirin)
- Acetaminophen (Anacin-3, Datril, Panadol, Phenaphen, Tylenol)
- Acetaminophen/Aspirin/Caffeine (Excedrin Migraine)
- NSAIDs—nonsteroidal antiinflammatory drugs
  - Nonprescription
    - Ibuprofen (Advil, Medipren, Motrin IB, Nuprin)

- Prescription
  - Naproxen (Naprosyn)
  - Naproxen sodium (Anaprox, Anaprox DS)
  - Mefenamic acid (Ponstel)
  - Tolfenamic acid (Tolfedine, Tolfine, Clotam)
  - Indomethacin (Indocin)
  - Flurbiprofen (Ansaid)
  - Meclofenamate sodium (Meclomen)
  - Ketorolac tromethamine (Toradol)

For the ingredients in nonprescription painkillers for migraine, see the chart at the end of this chapter.

Aspirin

How It Works. Aspirin often is used as the first-line painkiller for infrequent migraine headaches that cause mild to moderate pain. Aspirin works to relieve pain in two ways. First, it acts on the brain's pain-control mechanism to raise the pain threshold and to reduce the perception of pain. Second, it has anti-inflammatory properties, and thus affects some of the mechanisms that make a headache hurt.

Aspirin usually is taken in tablet form in the United States, although it is commonly used in liquid and effervescent form in other countries. These forms have the advantage of getting into the bloodstream faster. Aspirin may also be combined with caffeine (e.g., Anacin, Maximum Strength Anacin), which helps speed its absorption from the stomach. The caffeine also acts as a mild cerebral stimulant, raising the level of certain brain chemicals.

Common Side Effects. Overuse of aspirin, as with other painkillers, may lead to rebound headache (see Chapter 21). Aspirin can cause gastrointestinal bleeding, and it should not be taken by anyone with a history of gastric ulcers or anyone who is on anticoagulants or other blood thinners. People who are sensitive to the drug may experience bronchospasms or skin reactions. Prolonged use, especially at high doses, may cause ringing in the ears (tinnitus) and deafness. Aspirin generally is not administered to children, as it is associated with a serious complication of certain viral illnesses, called Reye's syndrome.

Acetaminophen

How It Works. Acetaminophen (known as paracetamol in Canada, Britain, and other countries) is an effective alternative for people who have infrequent, mild to moderate migraine headaches but who cannot take aspirin. Acetaminophen, like aspirin, raises the pain threshold, but it does not have anti-inflammatory properties. Thus it affects the perception of pain, but does not really affect the processes responsible for head pain.

Like aspirin, acetaminophen usually is taken by tablet, but faster-acting liquid forms are available for adults and children. Acetaminophen may be combined with caffeine, e.g., Excedrin Migraine (FDA approved to treat mild to moderate migraines) or Extra Strength, to improve its absorption from the stomach.

Common Side Effects. Overuse of acetaminophen, as with other painkillers, may lead to rebound headache (see Chapter 21). Overdosage of acetaminophen may cause liver damage that may not show up for four to six days.

Nonsteroidal Anti-inflammatory Drugs (NSAIDs)

How They Work. The NSAIDs, one type of which now is available over the counter under various brand names, have been highly successful in treating moderate to severe migraine. They are often tried as a drug of first choice because they have fewer short-term side effects than stronger drugs and do not have the potential for abuse that opiates do.

NSAIDs share aspirin's dual action as an anti-inflammatory and a pain reliever. NSAIDs generally are more expensive than aspirin, but may be more effective than aspirin for severe migraines.

Many varieties of NSAIDs are available. All NSAIDs are similar in their efficacy, but patients respond to them very differently. Choosing the right one is a matter of trial and error, balancing the person's response and the side effects seen. Often-used drugs for migraine are the prescription NSAIDs naproxen (Naprosyn) and naproxen sodium (Anaprox). Other NSAIDs known to be useful for migraineurs are mefenamic acid (Ponstel) and tolfenamic acid (Tolfedine, Tolfene, Clotam). Some physicians also have used an injectable NSAID, ketorolac tromethamine (Toradol), and found it to be stronger and faster-acting than other NSAIDs.

Common Side Effects. Among the possible side effects of NSAIDs are gastrointestinal discomfort and bleeding, edema, water retention, increased blood pressure, nausea, ringing in the ears, vertigo, and kidney damage. People who are hypersensitive to aspirin, particularly if they are asthmatics, generally should avoid NSAIDs as well.

A Special Note About Simple Analgesics

All drugs—whether sold by prescription or over the counter—are powerful substances that must be taken with care. Even "simple" aspirin can have significant side effects if taken improperly or by people who should not be using it because of their medical histories.

Be sure to consult your physician about the use of all drugs, even simple over-the-counter painkillers. Never exceed the dosage recommended on the label of a nonprescription painkiller without your doctor's permission. Follow your physician's directions carefully. This is especially true for prescription NSAIDs, which really are not "simple" at all and which can have significant side effects if not properly used.

Combination Analgesics

Combination Analgesics for Migraine

- Barbiturate compounds (Esgic, Esgic-Plus, Fioricet, Fiorinal, Phrenilin, Phrenilin Forte)
- Muscle relaxant compounds (Norgesic, Norgesic Forte)
- Narcotic compounds
  - Oxycodone hydrochloride preparations (Percocet, Percodan, Percodan-Demi, Roxicet, Roxicet 5/500, Roxiprin, Tylox)
  - Dihydrocodeine bitartrate preparations (Synalgos-DC)
  - Hydrocodone bitartrate preparations (Bancap HC, Co-Gesic, Dolacet, Hydrocet, Hy-Phen, Lorcet-HD, Lorcet Plus, Lortab 2.5/500, Lortab 5/500, Lortab 7.5/500, Lortab ASA, Vicodin, Vicodin ES, Zydone)
  - Propoxyphene preparations (Darvocet N 50/100, Darvon Compound-65, Dolene AP-65, Wygesic)
  - Codeine preparations (Codalan, Empirin with codeine, Fiorinal with codeine, Phenaphen with codeine, Phenaphen-650 with codeine, Tylenol with codeine)

For the specific components of these combination analgesics, see the chart at the end of this chapter.

How They Work. Combination drugs may be the most commonly prescribed drugs for acute migraine pain. They contain aspirin or acetaminophen along with a muscle relaxant, a barbiturate, and/or a narcotic analgesic. They may also contain caffeine to improve absorption from the stomach.

Common Side Effects. All combination drugs have a high potential to cause rebound headaches if they are overused. In addition, too frequent use of narcotic combinations may lead to dependence.

All may cause dizziness and fatigue; narcotic compounds may also cause depression or constipation. They may also have the side effects associated with the aspirin or acetaminophen that is part of the compound.

Specific Antimigraine Drugs

Specific Antimigraine Drugs Used for Acute Migraine

- Ergotamine tartrate (Cafergot, Wigraine, Ergostat)
- Isometheptene mucate combinations (Midrin, Isocom)
- Dihydroergotamine (DHE-45)
- Sumatriptan (Imitrex)

Ergotamine Tartrate

How They Work. Ergot compounds, derived from a fungus that grows on rye, have long been used as a primary choice for the treatment of acute migraine. Ergotamine tartrate affects several systems thought to be directly involved in migraine: it affects the serotonin system, constricts blood vessels, and combats inflammation. Ergot drugs often are prescribed as a preventative for menstrual migraine, to be used only around the time of menstruation. (See Chapter 17).

Common Side Effects. Ergotamine can cause nausea or make it worse. When used more than twice a week, ergotamine may cause rebound headaches. In rare cases overuse of ergots may lead to a condition called ergotism. (See Chapter 21.)

Isometheptene Mucate Combinations

How They Work. Isometheptene mucate, in combination with acetaminophen and dichloralphenazone, is often used in place of ergotamine or combination drugs to treat acute migraine. It is often used in children and in people who cannot tolerate ergotamine. Although its action in the body is different from ergotamine's, it works on the processes responsible for head pain by constricting blood vessels.

Common Side Effects. The most common side effect people report is dizziness. The drug should not be taken more than three times a week.

Dihydroergotamine (DHE-45)

How It Works. DHE is an alkaloid of ergot. It is a powerful agent for use in cases of severe migraine, often relieving pain within thirty minutes to four hours. Unlike most other acute drugs, DHE works even when the headache pain is at its height.

DHE is thought to work on the serotonin system of the brain and blood vessels. It affects the way blood flows in the head and neck, constricting blood vessels and reducing inflammation around them as a result of its effects on serotonin action.

When given in the hospital or in an emergency department, DHE is typically given intravenously. For out-of-hospital use physicians can inject it subcutaneously or intramuscularly, and patients can use an autoinjectable dose or DHE suppositories (which are not commercially manufactured but which can be easily compounded by a pharmacist). An intranasal (inhaled) form of DHE is also in use. Because DHE can be self-administered, someone with a severe migraine attack may be able to avoid a trip to the emergency room.

Common Side Effects. Side effects are common with DHE, but few are serious enough to stop the treatment. Many patients experience pain or burning around the injection site. Most people take an antinausea drug about twenty to thirty minutes before taking DHE, because DHE can cause nausea or vomiting. Other common side effects are drowsiness, body aches, and fatigue or diarrhea.

Some people experience temporary worsening of their headache within thirty minutes of taking DHE. It is important to be aware of this possibility so you won't become alarmed if it happens. In most cases this side effect lasts no more than ten to twenty minutes, and then your pain begins to decrease significantly.

Your physician will have to decide if DHE is right for you. Because DHE constricts blood vessels in the body as well as in the head, it may be inappropriate for some patients with angina or other heart conditions. In addition, pregnant women and people who are hypersensitive to ergots should not take DHE.

DHE does not result in physical dependence, but some researchers believe that using more than three injections a day, or more than five in a week, may lead to rebound headache. (See Chapter 21).

Triptans

The major advance in the treatment of migraine in recent years has been the arrival of the triptans as a "designer class" of medication. Unlike earlier medications that were developed or discovered by a trial-and-error process, the triptans were designed to interact with specific serotonin receptors in the brain that are known to be involved in a migraine attack. These medications stop migraine as it occurs. They are so miraculous in their effects for many patients that a guide for patients is in order, since the number of available triptans is multiplying rapidly.

How They Work. All of the triptans currently available share a common mode of action. They activate specific types of serotonin receptors on nerves and blood vessels and in so doing turn off inflammation and shrink swollen blood vessels believed to contribute to migraine pain. However, all of the triptans also narrow coronary arteries and cannot be used by persons who have blood vessel or heart disease or who are at high risk for heart disease, which is a disadvantage.

As doctors and patients look at the triptans, they try to match the individual's needs to the medication. Three of the triptans have fast action-sumatriptan (Imitrex), zolmitriptan (Zomig), and rizatriptan (Maxalt). One of the triptans, naratriptan (Amerge), is slower to act but its effects last longer. Naratriptan has fewer side effects, but all constrict arteries the same. Patients should not switch triptans within the same day. So, if one triptan fails to relieve a headache, a patient cannot rescue with another triptan. Sumatriptan, however, comes in multiple forms (injection, nasal spray, and tablet), and a patient can switch forms if needed.

Side Effects. A problem with triptans is that the headache may return hours after initial successful treatment. Some triptans show lower headache recurrence rates and longer duration of effect. This can be important for patients who have more prolonged migraine attacks. Now patients and their doctors can pick their medication based both on the nature of their migraine and its variability, and on the qualities of the triptans, their efficacy, available forms, side effects, consistency, and duration of effect.

On the Triptan Horizon: Several new triptans, such as eletriptan (Relpax), frovatriptan, and almotriptan, are in the development or approval process. Ask your physician or the American Council for Headache Education for the latest information on their status.

Major Tranquilizers

Major Tranquilizers for Acute Migraine Pain

- Chlorpromazine (Thorazine)
- Prochlorperazine (Compazine)
- Trifluoperazine (Stelazine)

How They Work. Major tranquilizers, or phenothiazines, act on a portion of the brain called the hypothalamus. They can help relieve the nausea as well as the pain of migraine, but they may "zonk you out" because they have very powerful effects.

Phenothiazines are administered as tablets, in suppositories, and in liquid forms. They are also given intravenously in the emergency department for people with severe migraine pain, especially when they are also experiencing severe stomach disturbances.

Common Side Effects. These drugs may cause sedation, dry mouth, drowsiness, and restlessness in some people. They also may occasionally cause the troublesome (although almost always temporary) side effects known as *extrapyramidal effects,* which include a variety of movement disturbances, such as involuntary grimaces or limb movements, and symptoms similar to those of parkinsonism.

Narcotics

Narcotics Prescribed for Acute Migraine Pain

- Propoxyphene (Darvon, Darvon-N, Dolene)
- Oxycodone hydrochloride (Roxicodone)
- Meperidine (Demerol, Penthadol)
- Hydromorphone (Dilaudid)
- Morphine (MSIR, M S Contin, Roxanol)
- Butorphanol tartrate (Stadol, Stadol NS)

How They Work. Narcotics, which act on the central nervous system's pain receptors to reduce the perception of pain, are highly effective in treating headaches that do not respond to other painkillers. But with the advent of DHE and sumatriptan, which act specifically on the serotonin system, narcotics are no longer the logical next step for people whose ergotamine or analgesics fail.

Common Side Effects. Over time regular use of narcotics can cause dependence and rebound headaches. They may also cause fatigue, dizziness, constipation, and depression. Butorphanol tartrate, an opioid agonist-antagonist available in a nasal spray, is not a controlled substance and may be somewhat less likely to lead to dependence. But it, too, must be used with caution.

Corticosteroids

Corticosteroids for Acute Migraine Pain

- Dexamethasone
- Prednisone

How They Work. Corticosteroids work to reduce inflammation. They may be effective in treating headaches in people who can't use ergotamine, DHE, or sumatriptan or whose headaches don't respond to these or other treatments.

Common Side Effects. When used regularly these drugs can cause significant physical changes, such as weight gain, water retention, high blood pressure, and gastrointestinal problems. To avoid these problems many physicians limit corticosteroid use to no more than once a month.

Minor Tranquilizers

Minor Tranquilizers Used for Acute Migraine Pain

- **Benzodiazepines**
  - Diazepam (Valium)
  - Alprazolam (Xanax)
  - Clorazepate (Tranxene, Tranxene-SD)

- Chlordiazepoxide (Librium, Libritabs)
- Lorazepam (Ativan)
▪ **Barbiturates**
- Phenobarbital (Solfoton)
▪ **Other Anxiolytics**
- Buspirone (BuSpar)

How They Work. Minor tranquilizers usually are not considered within the primary arsenal of treatments for acute migraine, but they can be used to raise the pain threshold, bring about relaxation and sleepiness, and reduce anxiety.

Common Side Effects. The benzodiazepines, when overused, are likely to cause dependence and require withdrawal under the care of a physician. They may also cause fatigue, dizziness, or sleepiness.

THE IMPORTANCE OF SLEEP

Sleep is part of the natural healing process when a migraine occurs. For many people with migraine, however, sleep is elusive once the headache sets in.

Migraineurs who can sleep recover better and with less medication than those who only rest or doze. Some physicians prescribe a short-acting benzodiazepine, such as 10 mg diazepam (Valium), as an adjunct to an ergot or other acute medication to help a patient relax enough to sleep. Benzodiazepines, however, must be used with care, because they can cause dependence if overused.

Some people who are particularly sensitive to caffeine may find that even the small amounts contained in certain ergot derivatives will interfere with their ability to sleep. Talk to your physician about this possibility. He or she may try you on another ergotamine preparation without caffeine before giving you an additional drug for sleeping.

TREATMENT OF AURA

Usually the aura of migraine is not specifically treated, because it ends quickly when the headache appears. Some patients, however, experience prolonged auras. For these patients, as well as for those with hemiplegic migraine and basilar migraine (see Chapter 5), in which the aura is accompanied by other neurological impairments, treatment has to address the aura as well as the pain, nausea, and malaise that follows it.

To stop the aura physicians may use sublingual nifedipine, carbon dioxide mixed with air or oxygen, amyl nitrite, or isoproterol.

For people with prolonged auras, beta blockers and ergot derivatives (such as the drugs Methysergide and Methergine, discussed in Chapter 14) usually are not used as first-choice preventive treatments. Some reports suggest that these agents may increase the risk of stroke for such patients.

Active Ingredients in Some Nonprescription Drugs Commonly Used for Migraine

Product Name	Aspirin	Acetaminophen	Caffeine	Ibuprofen	Other Active Ingredients
Aspirin	325 mg	0	0	0	0
Advil	0	0	0	200	0
Anacin	400 mg	0	32 mg	0	0
Anacin, Maximum Strength	500 mg	0	32 mg	0	0
Anacin-3	0	325 mg	0	0	0
Anacin-3, Maximum Strength	0	500 mg	0	0	0
Ascriptin	325 mg	0	0	0	Maalox 50 mg (antacid)
Bufferin	325 mg	0	0	0	Calcium carbonate, magnesium oxide, and magnesium carbonate as buffers

Medication					
Bufferin, Extra Strength	500 mg	0	0	0	Calcium carbonate, magnesium oxide, and magnesium carbonate as buffers
Cope	421 mg	0	32 mg	0	antacids
Datril, Extra Strength	0	500 mg	0	0	0
Excedrin PM	0	500 mg	0	0	Diphenhydramine citrate (mild sedative)
Excedrin, Aspirin Free	0	500 mg	65 mg	0	0
Excedrin, Ex. Strength, or Migraine	250 mg	250 mg	65 mg	0	0
Ecotrin	325 mg	0	0	0	0
Ecotrin, Maximum Strength	500 mg	0	0	0	0
Empirin	325 mg	0	0	0	0

Product Name	Aspirin	Acetaminophen	Caffeine	Ibuprofen	Other Active Ingredients
Medipren	0	0	0	200 mg	0
Midol	454 mg	0	32.4 mg	0	cinnamedrine (antispasmodic)
Motrin IB	0	0	0	200 mg	0
Nuprin	0	0	0	200 mg	0
Panadol	0	500 mg	0	0	0
Percogesic	0	325 mg	0	0	phenyltoloxamine citrate 30 mg (mild sedative)
Phenaphen	0	325 mg	0	0	0
Tylenol	0	325 mg	0	0	0
Tylenol, Extra Strength	0	500 mg	0	0	0
Vanquish	227 mg	194 mg	33 mg	0	antacids

	Active Ingredients in Some Prescription Combination Analgesics Commonly Used for Migraine			
Product Name	Barbiturate/Muscle Relaxant/Narcotic Ingredient	Aspirin	Acetaminophen	Caffeine
Barbiturate Compounds				
Esgic	butalbital 50 mg	0	325 mg	40 mg
Esgic-Plus	butalbital 50 mg	0	500 mg	40 mg
Fioricet	butalbital 50 mg	0	325 mg	40 mg
Fiorinal	butalbital 50 mg	325 mg	0	40 mg
Phrenilin	butalbiltal 50 mg	0	325 mg	0
Phrenilin Forte	butalbital 50 mg	0	650 mg	0
Muscle Relaxant Compounds				
Norgesic	orphenadrine citrate 25 mg	385 mg	0	30 mg
Norgesic Forte	orphenadrine citrate 50 mg	770 mg	0	60 mg
Narcotic Compounds				
Bancap HC	hydrocodone bitartrate 5 mg	0	500 mg	0

Product Name	Barbiturate/Muscle Relaxant/Narcotic Ingredient	Aspirin	Acetaminophen	Caffeine
Codalan	codeine: #1, 8 mg #2, 15 mg #3, 30 mg	0	500 mg	30 mg
Co-Gesic	hydrocodone bitartrate 5 mg	0	325 mg	0
Darvocet-N 50/100	propoxyphen napsylate 50/100 mg	0	325 mg	0
Darvon Compound-65	propoxyphene hydrochloride 65 mg	389 mg	0	32.4 mg
Dolacet	hydrocodone bitartrate 5 mg	0	500 mg	0
Dolene AP-65	propoxyphene hydrochloride 65 mg	0	650 mg	0
Empirin with Codeine	codeine: #2, 15 mg #3, 30 mg #4, 60 mg	325 mg	0	0
Fiorinal with Codeine	codeine 30 mg butalbital 50 mg	325 mg	0	40 mg
Hydrocet	hydrocodone bitartrate 5 mg	0	500 mg	0

Hy-Phen	hydrocodone bitartrate 5 mg	0	500 mg	0
Lorcet-HD	hydrocodone bitartrate 5 mg	0	500 mg	0
Lorcet Plus	hydrocodone bitartrate 7.5 mg	0	650 mg	0
Lortab 2.5/500, 5/500, 7.5/500	hydrocodone bitartrate 2.5/5/7.5 mg	0	500 mg	0
Lortab ASA	hydrocodone bitartrate 5 mg	500 mg	0	0
Percocet	oxycodone hydrochloride 5 mg	0	325 mg	0
Percodan	oxycodone hydrochloride 4.5 mg oxycodone terephthalate 0.38 mg	325 mg	0	0
Percodan-Demi	oxycodone hydrochloride 2.25 mg oxycodone terephthalate 0.19 mg	325 mg	0	0

Product Name	Barbiturate/Muscle Relaxant/Narcotic Ingredient	Aspirin	Acetaminophen	Caffeine
Phenaphen with Codeine	codeine: #2, 15 mg #3, 30 mg #4, 60 mg	0	325 mg	0
Phenaphen-650 with Codeine	codeine 30 mg	0	650 mg	0
Roxicet	oxycodone hydrochloride 5 mg	0	325 mg	0
Roxicet 5/500	oxycodone hydrochloride 5 mg	0	500 mg	0
Roxiprin	oxycodone hydrochloride 4.5 mg oxycodone terephthalate 0.38 mg	325 mg	0	0
Synalgos-DC	dihydrocodeine bitartrate 16 mg	356.4 mg	0	30 mg
Tylenol with Codeine	codeine: #1, 7.5 mg #2, 15 mg #3, 30 mg #4, 60 mg	0	300 mg	0

Tylox	oxycodone hydrochloride 5 mg	0	500 mg	0
Vicodin	hydrocodone bitartrate 5 mg	0	500 mg	0
Vicodin ES	hydrocodone bitartrate 7.5 mg	0	750 mg	0
Wygesic	propoxyphene hydrochloride 65 mg	0	650 mg	0
Zydone	hydrocodone bitartrate 5 mg	0	500 mg	0

CHAPTER 14

Medications for Migraine: Prevention and Case Studies

For people who have four to six or more migraines a month, or who do not have much luck with acute medications, preventive therapies may bring some measure of relief.

Most preventive drugs are taken daily, whether headache is present or not. With long-term administration many drugs may lose their efficacy (see Chapter 12). For this reason physicians usually prefer to put the patient on a different drug after six months or a year. Often they will wait a short while before switching the person to another preventive drug, to see if the headache condition has improved sufficiently to warrant using acute drugs alone.

Be sure to follow your doctor's instructions carefully for when and how to take your medications. Never change your dosage or stop your medication without discussing it first with your doctor.

Types of Preventive Drugs for Migraine

- Beta Blockers
- Calcium Channel Blockers
- Antiserotonin Agents
- Anticonvulsants
- Antidepressants

All preventive drugs for migraine have side effects—some mild, some significant. Each person reacts differently, sometimes to different drugs within the same class of drugs. The greatest challenge in prescribing preventive agents is to find one that gives an individual patient the maximum benefits with the least troublesome side effects.

A COMMON MISUNDERSTANDING ABOUT MIGRAINE PREVENTIVES

All the drugs currently in use to prevent migraine were originally created to treat conditions other than migraine. For this reason some migraineurs have misconceptions about why their physicians prescribe certain drugs.

One woman, for example, complained that "doctors don't really listen; they just think you're depressed and put you on a tricyclic." It is important to note that drugs such as Prozac, Zoloft, and the tricyclics are *not* prescribed chiefly for their antidepressant qualities. They are prescribed because they seem to affect the complex neurochemicals that are involved in making a migraine.

Similarly, you don't take a beta blocker or calcium channel blocker because the physician thinks your migraines are caused by heart problems or high blood pressure. These drugs affect the blood vessels, and blood vessels play a significant role in migraine disorder.

PREVENTIVE DRUGS USED FOR MIGRAINE

While many drugs are used to treat migraine, only four are FDA approved for such use: divalproex sodium (Depakote), propranolol (Inderal), timolol (Blocadren), and methysergide (Sansert).

Beta Blockers

Beta Blockers Used for Migraine Prevention

- Propranolol (Inderal)
- Nadolol (Corgard)
- Atenolol (Tenormin)
- Timolol (Blocadren)
- Metoprolol (Lopressor)

How They Work. Beta blockers are the drugs most often used for preventing migraine. According to recent research they are 60 to 80 percent effective in reducing the frequency of migraine attacks by half or more.

Scientists are not sure exactly how beta blockers work, but they inhibit the action of certain chemicals inside and outside of the brain, some of which affect blood pressure and pulse. Response to beta blockers is highly individual, and physicians may try larger doses or switch you to another beta blocker if you don't respond.

Common Side Effects. Beta blockers may cause fatigue, depression, sleep problems, weight gain, decreased tolerance for exercise, edema, dizziness, memory disturbance, hallucinations, gastrointestinal problems, slowed heartbeat, or impotence. People with congestive heart failure, asthma, or insulin-dependent diabetes should not take beta blockers.

Calcium Channel Blockers

Calcium Channel Blockers Used for Migraine Prevention

- Verapamil (Calan, Isoptin)
- Nifedipine (Procardia)
- Diltiazem (Cardizem)

How They Work. Calcium channel blockers block the release of serotonin and prevent calcium from entering certain cells. These actions have a wide range of effects on the cardiovascular system and appear to prevent inflammation of the blood vessels in the head. It may take two months or more of treatment before the drug begins to show positive effects.

In addition to the drugs mentioned here, flunarizine, a calcium channel blocker not available in the United States, also has been shown to be effective in preventing migraine.

Common Side Effects. In some people calcium channel blockers may cause constipation, edema, nausea, fatigue, low blood pressure, flushing, dizziness, or headache (including migraine).

Antiserotonin Agents

Antiserotonin Agents Used for Migraine Prevention

- Methysergide (Sansert)
- Methylergonovine maleate (Methergine)
- Cyproheptadine (Periactin)
- Ergotamine tartrate with phenobarbital and alkaloids of belladonna (Bellergal)

How They Work. These drugs interfere with the action of serotonin, a brain chemical that plays a major role in causing migraine. Sansert is the oldest approved migraine preventive and used to be considered the frontline treatment for migraine. Methergine replaces ergonovine, an older drug no longer available. Periactin, an antihistamine, is most often used for children with migraine and for hormonally related migraine. Bellergal is most likely to be used as a preventive agent by women with migraine during the days around the menstrual period, since ergotamine tartrate can cause rebound problems if used continuously.

Common Side Effects. In some cases these drugs may cause weight gain, sedation, fluid retention, urinary retention, constriction of the blood vessels, nausea, or cramping.

In rare cases long-term use of methysergide can produce fibrous changes in and around the heart, lungs, or kidneys. To prevent this problem patients using the drug are carefully followed and are taken off the drug for a month after every six months of use.

Anticonvulsants

Anticonvulsants Used for Migraine Prevention

- Divalproex sodium (Depakote)
- Phenytoin (Dilantin)
- Carbamazepine (Tegretol)
- Gabapentin (Neurontin)
- Lamotrigine (Lamictal)

How They Work. These drugs, ordinarily used to prevent seizures in epileptic patients, have been used to treat children with migraine as well as adults who have not responded to other therapies.

Common Side Effects. In some people anticonvulsants may cause dizziness, nausea, sedation, gastrointestinal disturbances, or temporary hair loss.

Antidepressants Used for Migraine Prevention

- Tricyclics
  - Nortriptyline (Aventyl, Pamelor)
  - Amitriptyline (Elavil, Endep)
  - Doxepin (Sinequan, Adapin)
  - Imipramine (Tofranil)
- MAO Inhibitors
  - Phenelzine (Nardil)
- Serotonin-uptake Inhibitors
  - Fluoxetine (Prozac)
  - Paroxetine (Paxil)
  - Sertraline (Zoloft)
  - Citalopram (Celexa)
- Atypical Antidepressants
  - Trazodone
  - Serzone
  - Wellbutrin
  - Effexor

How They Work. These drugs affect the serotonin receptors in the central nervous system. It is this action, not their antidepressant effects, that makes them effective in treating migraine.

The tricyclic antidepressants sometimes are used in combination with a beta blocker or calcium channel blocker. MAO inhibitors are used chiefly in cases where the migraineur has not been helped by other therapies, and may be used in conjunction with tricyclics. Although the serotonin-uptake inhibitors affect certain of the neurochemicals involved in migraine, it is not clear whether they are especially helpful to migraineurs. A new serotonin-uptake inhibitor, Paroxetine hydrochloride (Paxil) recently was approved for use in the U.S. and may be prescribed for some migraineurs.

Two other types of antidepressants are not much used for migraine prevention. Lithium carbonate, an antidepressant often used in treating bipolar disorder (manic-depressive syndrome), has been used to treat an uncommon type of migraine that occurs with the frequency of cluster headaches. The tetracyclic antidepressants, such as maprotiline (Ludiomil), have not been established as helpful in preventing migraine.

Common Side Effects. The most common side effects of the tricyclics are dry mouth and eyes, constipation, weight gain, and fatigue.

MAO inhibitors require a special diet and restriction of other medications. In some cases they may cause weight gain and sudden increases in blood pressure.

In some people the serotonin uptake inhibitors may cause restlessness, weight gain, sleep problems, and agitation. Desyrel may cause fatigue or painful, prolonged erections in men.

MIGRAINE RELIEF WITH THE HELP OF MEDICATION: THREE CASE STUDIES

Denise A.

Denise A. can't remember when she didn't have headaches. "I remember Mother giving me baby aspirin when I was playing with friends in the backyard," she said.

The first time Denise had a headache that didn't respond to baby aspirin occurred when she was eight years old, while her parents were out and her older sister was babysitting. Denise lay on the couch for several hours holding her head and crying. Although it was a frightening experience for her and for her eleven-year-old sister, everyone shrugged it off as "just a headache."

Denise experienced bad headaches all through high school and college. She treated them with aspirin, often downing six or seven tablets within a two-hour period. A night's sleep or rest in a dark room would help the aspirin work. Otherwise the headaches remained. The attacks came more frequently when she traveled, when she ate a lot of cheese, and when she stayed up late studying. Because she had experienced these headaches most of her life, she didn't know life could be different—until she was pregnant the first time.

"The best part of being pregnant was that I didn't have any headaches," said Denise. Thinking that pregnancy might have cured her headaches, she was dismayed when they returned with a vengeance after her twins were born. She managed to function enough to care for her babies, but when her husband returned home from work, she turned everything over to him and went to bed. Often she found herself having to hire a sitter to watch the children. Extremely discouraged because she was missing so much of the joy of watching her babies develop, she decided she had to let her family physician know about her problems.

"I was scared to death to tell him," she said. "Not because I thought I had a brain tumor or something but because I really expected him to tell me to 'just relax' and they would go away." She feared that he would assume that she was a bad manager or too much of a perfectionist, or that he would say she needed to do something about her "Type A" personality.

When Denise finally admitted to her physician that her headaches made it difficult for her to function and to be the kind of mother she wanted to be to her babies, her doctor's response put her immediately at ease. "Oh, Denise, I'm sorry," he said. "We don't want that. I think we can do something about those headaches." The physician explained that his mother had experienced migraine headaches, and he felt a real responsibility to help anyone who was in a similar situation.

Although the doctor was fairly certain Denise had migraine, he ordered an MRI to rule out other problems. When the results showed no other problems, he started her on a low daily dose of Inderal.

"I experienced a little diarrhea the first week or so, but, hey, I didn't have headaches anymore, and that was wonderful," said Denise. The diarrhea subsided and the headaches didn't return.

Denise has not had a migraine for nearly a year. She does sometimes experience a mild tension-type headache—the kind that responds to a couple of Tylenol.

Wendy K.

Wendy K. began having migraine when she reached puberty and started menstruating. When most girls were complaining of mild—or even severe—menstrual cramps but were able to continue attending school, Wendy was home in bed for three days with a blinding migraine. For thirty years she has had migraine attacks nearly every month.

Wendy has tried everything from biofeedback and massage to beta blockers and painkillers. In her early years her experiences were extremely frustrating because she felt she got the brush-off from physicians. She heard such comments as "What you need is a husband" or "What you need is to have another baby," implying that her pain was the result of an empty or unfulfilled life.

When she finally found a physician who took her problem seriously, she was prescribed a variety of medications, including ergotamine tartrate for seven days around her periods. The ergotamine has brought her some relief, but only when she takes it faithfully according to the schedule.

In conjunction with her medication Wendy practices relaxation exercises and has regular sessions with a massage therapist. She still spends at least one day in bed each month because of migraine, but she has been able to use the resources of medication and relaxation exercises to lessen the impact.

As she approaches midlife, she looks forward to menopause, hoping that it will finally bring permanent relief.

Joe B.

Joe B. began getting headaches early in his teens. At fifty-seven, he still experiences two headaches a week, though not all of them are migraines. His migraine attacks last from twelve to twenty-four hours, and he usually experiences them once every two or three weeks.

Joe handled his migraine attacks on his own with fistfuls of aspirin until the aspirin caused a bleeding ulcer. "My GI doctor advised me to be more cautious about aspirin products, and he prescribed Fioricet," said Joe. "That worked fairly well, though it didn't always take away the pain."

A year ago the doctor prescribed Midrin for Joe. "That works reasonably well, and the only side effects are that it makes me a little bit tired," he said.

Joe said he considers himself one of the lucky ones because he can eventually get rid of the migraine with relatively mild medication. But he still wakes up in the middle of the night with migraine when the weather changes. And if he's even an hour late eating lunch, he can count on having a migraine. He usually feels lethargic and a little nauseous before the head pain hits him.

Joe's brother and father both have migraine. His brother tried biofeedback. "He was indifferent about biofeedback, but he takes Inderal to prevent migraine," said Joe.

Joe said he's not ready for Inderal. "I'm tempted to try biofeedback, though," he added.

CHAPTER 15

Nondrug Therapies

In recent years a number of what might once have been considered unorthodox approaches to treating illness and pain have gained credibility in the medical community. Some are becoming part of the physician's arsenal of management strategies for people with migraine. Many headache clinics, for example, offer biofeedback as a option. And it is not unusual for physicians to place a patient on a treatment plan that includes some kind of drug therapy but also involves a regimen of exercise, proper nutrition, and relaxation techniques.

Some people say they receive significant help from one or another of the nondrug therapies discussed in this chapter. Responses to these therapies, however, are highly individual. Taking a long walk in the brisk fall air may help one person but may trigger a migraine in another. Self-hypnosis may dramatically decrease the pain one person experiences, while another may not be a good subject for hypnosis. Relaxation, like exercise, is good for a migraineur's overall well-being, but coming down too quickly from a stressful situation can sometimes trigger a migraine.

The only way to know if a nondrug therapy will work for you is to try it. But it's not a good idea to abandon your medications while you do so. For most people medications and nondrug therapies work hand in hand. If nondrug therapies are successful, they may allow you to take medications less often and in smaller doses.

Be sure to let your physician know about any nondrug therapies you are trying. The physician will want to monitor the effects and take them into account when prescribing medications.

TREATMENT OR PLACEBO?

Some of the nondrug therapies discussed in this chapter, such as biofeedback and progressive muscle relaxation, have been rigorously evaluated and found to be effective for a large number of migraineurs. Others, however, are more like folk remedies: there are lots of anecdotes about how well they work, but little medical evidence to prove their value. Some scientists believe that many nonmedical remedies act as placebos—treatments that have no specific value but that seem to help the body mobilize its own curative powers.

In a practical sense, whether these therapies actually treat the migraine or act as placebos is irrelevant. If they work for you, that's great.

Be suspicious, however, if someone offers you an expensive form of nonmedical therapy. People with chronic illnesses often fall under the influence of spurious practitioners who prey on the person's hope for a cure.

One woman, for example, went in for a visit to a "holistic healer" and found herself writing a check for more than $1,500 at the end of the visit. The vitamins and dietary restrictions he prescribed proved to be worthless—although she tried her best to believe they helped her, to justify the size of her investment!

Another woman went to someone who claimed to be a psychologist and who charged her more than $2,000 to pass a probe over her head and neck to "evaluate" her pain. "He was a complete con artist," the woman said.

Types of Nondrug Therapies

- Relaxation Methods
  - Biofeedback training
  - Progressive muscle relaxation
  - Hypnosis and self-hypnosis
  - Yoga
  - Autogenic training
  - Creative visualization
- Nutritional regimens
- Exercise
- Psychotherapy
- Physiological Methods
  - Oxygen therapy
  - Carbon dioxide therapy
  - Massage therapy
  - Acupuncture/acupressure
  - TENS (transcutaneous electrical nerve stimulation)
  - Hot or cold compresses
  - Osteopathy or chiropractic
  - Clinical ecology
  - Feverfew
  - Fish oil
  - Magnesium

Relaxation Methods

Relaxation methods are commonly prescribed as an adjunct to medical treatments for migraine. The type of relaxation method used does not seem to be important. Studies show that most methods are equally effective for migraine patients who learn to do them correctly and who practice them regularly. Therefore, you should choose a technique that appeals to you and that you will be able to perform correctly, with success, on your own.

Some experts on migraine think that regardless of the particular relaxation techniques migraine patients use, the significance of each technique is that patients shift from feeling controlled by events beyond their power to feeling like they are in control. Since people with migraine often feel controlled by their migraines, taking charge of their bodies through various relaxation methods returns to them a sense of control over their own lives and bodies.

Biofeedback Training

Lou W. is a thirty-two-year-old full-time student and free-lance writer. She began getting migraines when she was twenty-one and usually went to the emergency department in her hometown and received a combination analgesic. "Within an hour or two I would be asleep," she said. "But the doctors were reluctant to keep me on the drug."

Lou received biofeedback training in 1987, and she said it continues to help her reduce her overall stress response. "When I feel aura or pain starting, I lie down in a quiet place, make my hands warm and my forehead cool," she said. "At least ninety percent of the time it stops my headache." She now has only about three migraine attacks a year. "I have a life now," she said.

Biofeedback training as a method of teaching relaxation is well accepted by many physicians who treat headache. During biofeedback training, with the help of special equipment that monitors certain indicators of physical tension, you learn to use relaxation techniques to control involuntary and unconscious physical processes related to stress. In this way you can actually teach yourself to raise your skin temperature, lower your blood pressure, and relax the muscles in your body. Once you have learned what it feels like to control these processes, you can bring yourself into a deep state of relaxation anywhere and anytime, without the help of the equipment.

People with migraine typically use the relaxation techniques they learn in biofeedback training at the first sign of migraine, hoping to stop the attack or lessen its effects. Some also use the techniques daily as a preventive measure to help reduce the physical effects of stress. There is some evidence to show that both uses can be helpful to some people.

Although it is possible to find books that use simple biofeedback techniques to help you learn how to relax, biofeedback works best when you learn it from a trained and qualified person, usually a psychiatrist or psychologist. Many migraineurs report moderate to good success with biofeedback when they receive proper training and use it in conjunction with their medications. In addition to the whole-body relaxation that results, the biofeedback demonstrates to them that they can have control over their bodies and, by extension, their lives. This sense of control is very important to migraineurs, who often feel overpowered by their illness.

For people with hypersensitive nervous systems, however, biofeedback training can be a nerve-wracking experience. Many training devices use audible warnings—a bell or a buzzer—to let you know when your skin temperature or other physical indicator shows you are tense. "I couldn't do biofeedback," said one woman. "The sounds of the machine telling me I wasn't relaxed would make me even more tense. So it was just counterproductive."

When biofeedback training works for someone with migraine, it appears to have long-lasting therapeutic benefits. Some studies show that significant treatment benefits persist for six to seven years following the training. Several studies also suggest that biofeedback training in conjunction with short-term psychotherapy is more effective than biofeedback training alone.

Progressive Muscle Relaxation

Insomniacs have long used progressive muscle relaxation as an alternative to counting sheep. People with migraine who learn the technique use it the way biofeedback-trained people use their relaxation techniques, to reduce the pain of a migraine or even to stop it at an early stage.

In progressive muscle relaxation you contract and relax the different muscle groups in your body, beginning with your toes and working up through your feet, calves, thighs, abdomen, chest, arms, hands, neck, face, and head. You contract each group of muscles, hold them in contraction for five to ten seconds, then slowly let go. As you progress from group to group, you feel the amount of unnecessary tension you hold in your body.

Many people report feeling deeply relaxed when they complete the cycle of contractions and relaxations, with their thoughts floating by pleasantly. Some people who try progressive muscle relaxation, however, report that they are unable to use the technique. They find themselves becoming more fidgety and anxious lying down concentrating on their muscles.

Hypnosis and Self-hypnosis

Some people consider hypnosis little more than a parlor trick, while others think of it as a mind-control technique with the power to make people do foolish or illicit acts against their will. For people who can get beyond these notions, however, hypnosis and self-hypnosis may be on a par with biofeedback training and progressive muscle relaxation as an acute-care strategy for migraine.

A qualified hypnotherapist (usually a physician, psychologist, or psychotherapist who has received special training in hypnosis) does not try to cure your migraines by planting suggestions that you won't have them anymore. That technique rarely works—and certainly not over the long term. Instead, he or she often will begin by talking with you about the reasons you want more control over your headaches and the treatments you are following. Then the hypnotherapist leads you into a trance state and gives suggestions to help increase your inner motivation to control your headaches and to use relaxation techniques to control headache pain.

After one or more such sessions the hypnotherapist then teaches you how to self-induce a hypnotic trance. He or she may suggest sentences for you to repeat during the trance to help you relax and control your pain. This process, called "autosuggestion," probably is less important than the effect of trance itself, which produces deep relaxation. Like the relaxation techniques learned in biofeedback training, a self-hypnotic trance has a significant effect on your body, even increasing blood circulation.

Although some people are not good subjects for hypnosis, virtually everyone knows what it feels like to go into a self-hypnotic state. You may "trance out" while driving your car on a long trip, for example. You may go into a hypnotic trance while staring at the floor indicators in an elevator or while performing some repetitive task. The hypnotherapist merely teaches you to harness your natural ability to enter a hypnotic state to help you manage your migraines.

If you want to experience self-hypnosis on your own, bookstores and record stores carry many self-hypnosis videos and audiotapes. Choose ones that have titles like "Learn to Relax" or "Reduce Stress." Often the tapes will include soft ocean and bird sounds under calming music. On video the sounds may be accompanied by views of the ocean or other nature scenes. A voice may give instructions about relaxation or may repeat positive, affirming sentences about life. "I am relaxed and happy and full of peace," one says.

These tapes are useful for some people. One woman said she uses a meditation tape of Pachelbel's *Canon in D,* a familiar and well-loved composition. "It doesn't have suggestions, and the beginning has ocean sounds and bird sounds that are kind of hokey; it works for me," she said. "I often put myself to sleep at night with it, and if I'm where I can use my earphones, I listen to the tape to relax whenever I feel a migraine coming on."

Yoga

Yoga is an ancient form of meditative exercise that creates a sense of relaxation and well-being. Unlike aerobics and other strenuous exercises, yoga is a gentle exercise that focuses on slow, fluid movements and stretches.

If you try yoga, look for a qualified teacher. He or she will help you ease into these exercises so that you do not inadvertently injure your neck or back and possibly trigger a migraine. A good teacher also can tell you which yoga postures (called *asanas*) are especially beneficial for the vascular system and the nervous system.

If you can't find a yoga teacher in your area, or if you want to see more of what yoga is like before you try it, there are a number of excellent yoga videos for beginners available in video stores and by mail.

Autogenic Training

Autogenic training is a relaxation method that combines a form of self-hypnosis with progressive relaxation. Founded in the 1930s by psychiatrist Johannes Schultz, the system consists of a series of twelve suggestions focusing on different parts of the body, which you repeat to yourself in a fixed order:

1. My right arm feels heavy and warm.
2. My left arm feels heavy and warm.
3. My right leg feels heavy and warm.
4. My left leg feels heavy and warm.
5. My abdomen feels relaxed and warm.
6. My chest feels relaxed and warm.
7. My heartbeat is steady and calm.
8. My breathing is deep and relaxed.
9. My back feels heavy and warm.
10. My shoulders feel heavy and warm.
11. My neck feels heavy and cool.
12. My head feels heavy and cool.

As you repeat each suggestion, your goal is to experience—not think about—the physiological sensation it evokes while you breathe slowly and deeply. For example, when you have mastered autogenic training, you should *feel* your arm get heavy and warm, not merely repeat the words to yourself, when you say the first suggestion.

Some migraineurs report that autogenic training induces a powerful state of relaxation. The technique is sometimes difficult to learn, and so it usually is best to study it with the help of someone (often a psychologist) adept at the practice.

Creative Visualization

In creative visualization you learn to combine a relaxation exercise with a mental image of yourself without a migraine. This exercise can be quite effective for some people, especially if it is practiced at the very start of the migraine pain.

It is easy to try creative visualization for yourself. Begin with some type of relaxation exercise, such as progressive muscle relaxation, or simply listen to some calming music you enjoy. Next, imagine yourself in a pleasant situation. If you enjoy entertaining, perhaps you might imagine yourself preparing a meal and dining with friends in your home. If you like to swim, imagine yourself in a warm, clear lake under a cloudless blue sky. Whatever the scene, imagine yourself feeling energetic and well. If you already have a headache, imagine yourself slowly rolling the pain up into a tiny ball and pulling it out of your body, then imagine yourself participating in some activity you enjoy—migraine free.

If you enjoy creative visualization, there are many excellent books available to help you learn more about the technique.

Nutritional Regimens

It makes good sense to change your diet to avoid foods you've identified as migraine triggers (see Chapter 6, "Migraine

Triggers"). Eating regularly and eating a well-balanced diet also makes good sense for maintaining a generally healthy body.

Some people go further, however, and adopt stringent diets that promise to eliminate migraines by eliminating "food allergies." Many times these diets require you to consume special vitamins or other nutritional supplements while placing restrictions on what you eat. The regimen may begin with an "elimination diet," which tries to eliminate all possible sources of food allergy, then adds back foods gradually to see which ones you tolerate well.

There is no published, peer-reviewed scientific evidence to support the idea that such nutritional regimens can improve migraine, and the idea that food allergies are widespread and the underlying cause of many headaches is highly controversial. Some people may find their migraine condition improves temporarily when they start a restrictive diet, but this may be because fad diets often banish common migraine triggers such as alcohol and junk food. In the long run restrictive diets (except under medical supervision) may be dangerous to your health, and you will most likely be disappointed by any diet or "miracle food" that promises to banish migraines from your life.

Exercise

Moderate exercise, like proper nutrition, should be a part of every person's life. It contributes to cardiovascular health, weight maintenance, and a general sense of fitness. Beyond that, exercise can reduce your levels of stress and can create a psychological sense of well-being. The "runner's high," a state caused by the release of brain chemicals called endorphins, occurs during other types of exercise as well. Endorphins are the body's natural pain relievers and tend to elevate the mood.

The relationship between exercise and migraine is not clear. Some people report that moderate exercise, such as a brisk walk or low-impact aerobics, on a regular basis reduces the frequency of their headaches. In at least one study a woman who taught aerobics reported that even exercising during the headache phase of a migraine could alleviate her pain.

Very few people, however, would choose exercise once the migraine has begun. Because many people find that head movement exacerbates the pain, they wouldn't consider taking a stroll, let alone playing a game of tennis during a migraine. Even *watching* a tennis game could intensify the pain.

A Canadian study of people on a program of regular exercise indicated that the exercise reduced the frequency, intensity, and duration of their attacks. Other studies have shown, however, that exercise often precedes and may even precipitate migraine attacks.

Keep track of your exercise patterns in your headache diary (see Chapter 10), then modify them based on what you discover about yourself. If exercise seems to help you, experiment to see whether increasing the frequency or duration of exercise makes a positive difference. If some forms of exercise seem to trigger your migraines, try switching to some other form of exercise.

Psychotherapy

Even though psychological factors are not responsible for causing migraine (see Chapter 2, "Myths About Migraine"), they sometimes play a role in a person's ability to manage migraine. For this reason, in addition to the physical and pharmacological approaches to migraine treatment, some people find that psychotherapy can be useful.

Psychotherapy is practiced by a number of different specialists. *Psychiatrists* are physicians who specialize in the treatment of mental and emotional disorders. *Clinical psychologists, licensed clinical social workers,* and *licensed professional counselors* have specialized training in how to help people understand and manage their emotions, behaviors, and relationships. Any of these professionals may be able to help you learn how to cope more successfully with your migraines and their effects on your life.

Although there are dozens of different schools of therapy,

the most important point is to find a therapist you're comfortable with, who understands the effects of migraine or chronic pain on your life, and who is an intelligent, compassionate person. (For more information on how to choose a psychotherapist, see Chapter 24.)

Physiological Methods

Physiological therapies try to act directly on the physical symptoms and causes of migraine. In this way they are similar to drug therapies; where they differ, however, is in the kinds of agents used. Sometimes the agents are folk remedies or nutritional supplements available without prescription and not subject to the rigorous testing for safety and efficacy required for ordinary pharmaceuticals. Other times they may be external treatments that are administered by a medical doctor or trained professional. Physiological methods vary widely in technique and in rates of success.

Be cautious when evaluating physiological methods. Unlike other nondrug therapies these usually involve techniques or substances that have the potential for harm if misused. You might be wise to discuss them with your physician before trying them. In addition, because these therapies sometimes are expensive, you should carefully weigh the potential expense of a therapy against the probability that it will bring you significant relief. Be especially cautious if someone claims that the therapy in question can "cure" migraine.

Oxygen Therapy

Because oxygen constricts blood vessels, it might seem logical that oxygen would help at least some migraine patients. Cluster headaches (see Chapter 5) often are successfully treated by having the patient breathe 100 percent oxygen. Yet when the same technique was tried on migraine patients, it failed to show results.

One researcher recently tried treating twenty-six migraine

patients in a hyperbaric oxygen chamber—that is, a special chamber in which patients breathe pure oxygen delivered at two or more times the normal atmospheric pressure. All but two of these patients experienced complete pain relief within minutes, and only two experienced any return of their pain during the hours after treatment.

This single study was far too limited to prove that hyperbaric oxygen is an effective treatment for migraine. In any event it is not a very practical treatment, since many hospitals do not have hyperbaric oxygen chambers, and administration of oxygen in this way is expensive and requires highly specialized and trained personnel.

Carbon Dioxide Therapy

Some people find that breathing into a paper bag during the aura of migraine will stop the aura's progression. The active ingredient in this treatment is carbon dioxide, which becomes concentrated in the exhaled air. In cases of prolonged aura or complicated migraine (see Chapter 5), a physician may administer a combination of carbon dioxide and oxygen to stop the aura.

The carbon dioxide works by dilating the blood vessels. If the headache has not yet begun, the carbon dioxide may prevent the pain as well as stop the aura. Using this method after head pain has begun, however, usually intensifies the pain.

Massage Therapy

For some people regular visits to a trained massage therapist can bring about deep relaxation both during and after the massage and can play a role in reducing the number and frequency of migraines. In some cases a session of massage therapy during a migraine attack may diminish the pain.

There are many different techniques for massage therapy. The most common is the full-body Swedish massage available at many health clubs and consisting of kneading, tapping, or otherwise manipulating muscles throughout the body. Some health clubs also offer a more vigorous sports massage, focused on muscles that have been severely taxed by weight lifting or fast-paced sports.

Other techniques you may encounter are neuromuscular therapy, whose practitioners focus on painful areas called "trigger points"; Trager bodywork, which can be performed when you are fully dressed and which consists of gentle rocking motions to relieve stress throughout the body; postural integration, whose practitioners believe that stress distorts the normal alignment of muscles, tissues, and bones and who use a variety of hand pressures to reestablish normal body alignment; rolfing, a sequence of sessions, some of which are quite strenuous, that cumulatively relieve skeletomuscular tension and the emotional blockage that rolfing practitioners believe is at the source of physical problems; reiki, a sequence of gentle massage techniques you are taught to perform for yourself; and pain-relief and relaxation techniques such as myotherapy and deep tissue massage.

If you want to try massage therapy for your migraines, look for a certified massage therapist or a physical therapist. If you have never had a massage before, look for someone who practices one of the gentler forms of massage therapy, and tell him or her that you want to start slowly and gently.

Not everyone is a good candidate for massage therapy, however. People with high blood pressure, circulatory or heart problems, cancer or serious infections, or who are prone to bleeding or blood clots should not have massage. Vigorous massage may not be advisable for people with inflammatory disorders such as rheumatoid arthritis, because some people note that too-strenuous massage damages their delicate tissues and leads to increased inflammation and pain.

Even if you do not seek out a massage therapist, having a spouse or friend gently rub your face and head may provide temporary relief from the excruciating pain of a migraine. When the pain and nausea of a full-blown migraine overtake Suzanne S., she finds that medication alone doesn't help. "I have to lie down in a dark room and have someone massage my head," she said. "After about forty-five minutes the pain and nausea begin to subside."

Acupuncture/Acupressure

Acupuncture and acupressure are ancient Chinese techniques for relieving pain and restoring health. In acupuncture, thin needles are inserted into the skin at specific points and rotated; acupressure uses the same principles, but uses fingertip pressure on the designated points instead of needles.

Acupuncture and acupressure have not generally proven to be of much value as a migraine preventive. Some individuals, however, report that they have found at least temporary relief from the pain of a migraine attack if they undergo acupuncture or acupressure during a headache. If acupuncture or acupressure seems to work for you, you might ask the acupuncturist to teach someone who lives with you how to administer acupressure. This alternative would alleviate the greatest obstacle to using acupuncture or acupressure for migraine relief: it is often inconvenient or impossible for a migraineur to get to an acupuncturist when a headache comes on.

TENS (Transcutaneous Electrical Nerve Stimulation)

Transcutaneous electrical nerve stimulation (TENS) is a method of treating chronic pain by administering small electrical shocks to the painful area. It is not clear how these treatments work to relieve pain, but some people find that they do provide temporary relief for severe pain, especially when the pain is localized.

Headache pain is not often treated using TENS, in part because TENS treatments can only be administered by qualified physical therapists using special equipment. Because it works only on the symptoms of pain, TENS has no role in preventive treatment of migraine.

Application of Hot or Cold Compresses

Almost by instinct people with migraine reach for the ice pack or the cloth with steaming hot water to relieve their head pain.

Traditionally experts have believed that since cold compresses constricted the blood vessels, they would decrease the dilation associated with the pain of migraine. Hot compresses, on the other hand, have been considered better for the relief of tension headaches because they relax the muscles. In fact, however, some migraineurs use heat; others use cold. Many like to alternate them.

Pharmacies offer many convenient devices to deliver hot or cold therapy, including reusable gel packs and moist heat pads. Some people with migraine also have reported getting some relief from hot showers or hot baths.

Osteopathy or Chiropractic

Berta R. is a thirty-four-year-old woman, a part-time student and former professional athlete. She poured money into a number of medical and nonmedical therapies that didn't work for her. But a chiropractor has helped her a great deal. "I started last January going three times a week. After about three months it really turned things around for me," she said.

Osteopathy and chiropractic may seem like logical places to seek migraine relief, since practitioners of these disciplines manipulate the bones and tissues in the back and neck. But because migraine originates from within the brain and not from the bones and muscles of the head and neck, chiropractic and osteopathy have proven to be of minimal value in the treatment of migraine.

Some migraineurs who try chiropractic or osteopathy do report receiving some relief from the pain of a migraine in progress or, less often, a reduction in the frequency or severity of their attacks. Others say they experience relief from back and neck discomfort and tension but get little help for the migraine itself.

If you decide to see an osteopath or chiropractor, be sure to ask them to work slowly and carefully around your neck and head area. Some migraineurs report that too-vigorous neck and cranial manipulation seems to bring on a migraine. In rare cases too-aggressive manipulation can lead to serious injury.

Clinical Ecology

Clinical ecologists are physicians (and sometimes other medical professionals, such as osteopaths) who treat "environmental illness"—a loosely defined term that includes a variety of symptoms including fatigue, headache, and digestive disorders. Environmental illness usually is attributed to the body's response to a wide variety of allergens and other toxins—from building materials that give off formaldehyde and other toxic vapors to antibiotics that disrupt the normal ecological balance of benign microbes living in the human intestines.

A clinical ecologist may run a battery of blood and other tests to evaluate your general health and specific sensitivities. He or she may put you on a nutritional regimen; may prescribe medications, herbs, or vitamins to treat conditions such as systemic *candida albicans* (yeast) infection or to correct other imbalances; give you shots or other treatments for common allergies such as reactions to dust, animal dander, or mold; advise you on ways to avoid exposure to household chemicals, perfumes, and other common irritants; and suggest lifestyle changes, such as quitting smoking, increasing exercise, or changing your work habits.

Although headache specialists acknowledge that environmental chemicals are migraine triggers for some of their patients, clinical ecology is a highly controversial field. Some physicians consider environmental illness an important and underdiagnosed condition that deserves serious research, while others consider it quackery. Often the treatments prescribed are expensive and include large numbers of herbs and supplements that are not reimbursable by insurance and have not undergone rigorous testing for safety and effectiveness. In addition the idea that environmental illness may be the root cause of migraine contradicts current research findings that migraine is a primary disorder caused by abnormalities in brain chemistry.

Some people do report at least a temporary improvement in their migraines when undergoing treatment by a clinical ecologist. These changes may be related to improved trigger management, to improvements in general health because of lifestyle changes, or even to the placebo effect. If you choose to try clinical ecology, be sure to let your primary physician or headache specialist know what treatments you are taking.

Feverfew

An herbal remedy used frequently in England as a treatment for migraine, feverfew is a member of the chrysanthemum family of flowering plants. For centuries the folk remedy has been used as a sedative, tonic, aromatic, and mild laxative.

A study at University Hospital in Nottingham, England, suggested that daily use of feverfew can significantly reduce the frequency of migraine headaches. The study included fifty-nine people who had experienced at least one migraine headache a month for a minimum of two years. They were divided into two groups. One group received a capsule of dried feverfew leaves; the other group received a capsule of dried cabbage leaves. At the end of the four-month study the group that received the feverfew reported having had 135 fewer migraines than the other group. Neither group knew whether they were receiving feverfew or cabbage.

Feverfew recently has been making converts in the United States. One problem, however, is that there is no standardization of the strength of herbs in herbal teas or other preparations, and most are not labeled to show their concentrations. The strength of feverfew preparations sold commercially in health-food stores varies considerably. If you want to try feverfew, try buying samples of several brands to see which, if any, works for you.

Fish Oil

Numerous studies have shown that dietary fish oils contain substances that affect the blood and the blood vessels. Some migraineurs who take the fish-oil capsules sold in pharmacies and health-food stores report that the fish oils seem to reduce the frequency and severity of their migraine attacks. There have been a few small studies that seem to support the claim.

Taking large doses of fish oil, however, is not advisable, and any such dietary supplements should receive your doctor's approval. If you decide to try this remedy, your doctor probably will advise you to take a low dose—one gram or less per day.

Magnesium

Several recent studies have noted that many people who experience migraine have low blood levels of magnesium. Magnesium is an important dietary mineral that affects the workings of many organs and systems in the body, including the blood vessels.

Some physicians have been using injections of magnesium for migraineurs who have not had success with other treatments, and clinical trials of a special form of oral magnesium (not generally available) as a possible migraine preventive may soon get under way.

Although this treatment has not yet been rigorously evaluated and is not widely accepted among headache experts, some migraineurs have decided to test it themselves by taking oral magnesium supplements purchased in health-food stores. Administering magnesium to yourself in this way can be dangerous and can cause many side effects. Mineral supplements should only be taken under a doctor's care.

A Scorecard on Nondrug Therapies				
Type of Therapy	Common adjunct to medical treatment	May be helpful	Rarely helpful or rarely used	Special caution urged
Biofeedback training		X		
Progressive muscle relaxation		X		
Hypnosis and self-hypnosis		X		
Yoga		X		
Autogenic training		X		
Creative visualization		X		
Nutritional regimens	X (e.g., regular meals, balanced diet, trigger management)			X (fad diets, supplements, highly restricted diets)

Type of Therapy	Common adjunct to medical treatment	May be helpful	Rarely helpful or rarely used	Special caution urged
Exercise	X			
Psychotherapy		X		
Oxygen therapy			X	
Carbon dioxide therapy		X (for prolonged aura)	X (for head pain in progress)	
Massage therapy		X		
Acupuncture/ acupressure			X	
TENS (transcutaneous electrical nerve stimulation)			X	
Hot or cold compresses	X			

Osteopathy or chiropractic			X		
Clinical ecology			X		
Feverfew		X			
Fish oil					X
Magnesium					X

CHAPTER 16

Self-Help

"It's important to get involved in your own treatment, to keep trying other things, although it's hard to do when you're feeling so sick. A lot of things I've worked out for my own treatment have been in spite of the doctors."

Self-help is an important component of learning to live a full life with migraine. Migraineurs consistently report that an active balance of self-help and medical help brings them the best relief.

Self-care alone can be dangerous if it is not balanced by accurate medical diagnosis and medical management. By the same token medical diagnosis and management of the problem will help only minimally if you don't take seriously your role in managing your care.

BASIC PRINCIPLES OF SELF-CARE

An important component of self-care for migraine is maintaining overall good health. That includes a regimen of moderate exercise, proper rest, and good nutrition. Because strenuous exercise can sometimes bring on migraine, it is important to find a type and level of exercise that works for you. That might be a walk around the block, swimming a few laps in a heated pool, or working out on a ski machine.

It also is important to maintain a regular sleep schedule as part of your basic regimen of self-care. Many migraineurs get headaches when they sleep more or less than usual. Try to set a regular bedtime and a regular time to wake up. Avoid the temptation to stay up later than usual and sleep in on weekends.

Getting proper nutrition makes good sense for maintaining a generally healthy body, and it can also help you avoid migraines connected with diet. Eat a well-balanced diet comprised of approximately 60 percent carbohydrates, 25 percent fat, and 15 percent protein. Avoid dietary triggers you've identified (see Chapter 6). Don't skip meals, since skipped meals will often bring on a migraine if you're susceptible, and avoid junk-food binges, which bring on migraines in many people.

Managing your care also includes making sure you understand the types of medicines you are taking and what they do for you. Too many people with migraine make such comments as "I have three different pills that I take at different stages of the pain, but I don't know what they are or what they do." Part of taking care of yourself is knowing what kinds of medications you're putting into your body.

A final important part of self-care is self-help. Beyond the drugs your doctor prescribes, beyond the nondrug therapies you use for relaxation, symptom relief, and prevention, there are any number of simple remedies you can try that may make your headaches more manageable. If you are in a headache support group (see Chapter 24), try swapping self-help ideas with group members. Chances are you'll find a few ideas that will work for you.

SELF-HELP REMEDIES

Self-help ideas are as varied as the people who develop them. The following are just a few ideas that work for some people; they may or may not work for you.

> "While I'm waiting for my medication to work, I sit in the bathroom, put my hair dryer on low heat, and let it blow on my throbbing temple. Sometimes I alternate with an ice pack."
>
> —Berta R.

> "I can't bear to take a shower when I have a migraine, but I get into the bathtub and gently pour warm water over my head."
>
> —Suzanne S.

> "If I don't have to go anywhere, I may put an ice pack on the back of my neck. Other times a heating pad on my back will help."
>
> —Ruthe R.

> "If I wake up with the start of a headache, any motion at all will start it pounding—and then there will be little I can do for it. So I always keep liquid Tylenol (acetaminophen) on my bedside table. I can take a dose without moving very much, then lie back down to sleep. Many people don't realize that you can buy acetaminophen in a liquid form for adults. If you don't see it, ask the pharmacist."
>
> —Barbara T.

> "When I first get a headache, I put a baseball cap on my head and tighten the headband. The pressure feels good and makes the pain more manageable."
>
> —David A.

"When I feel a headache coming on, I take two No Doz. The caffeine in it seems to work better than just having a cup of coffee, and I can often stave off a headache that way."

—Heidi L.

"Weather changes often give me severe migraines that nothing really seems to help. But I can sometimes prevent them by taking one dose of Sudafed when I start feeling pressure around my eyes. If one dose doesn't work, I stop there and try something else."

—Lynne C.

"If synthetic odors seem to trigger your migraines, keep houseplants around. To combat low-level odors of formaldehyde, which can come from particle board, plywood, and foam insulation in new houses, upholstery on new furniture, or new synthetic carpeting, keep spider plants, rhapis, dracaena, and sansevieria. To combat the benzene from cigarettes, detergents, inks, and oils, use hedera and spathiphyllum. Chrysanthemums will help protect against trichlorethylene, which is given off by varnishes, lacquers, and glues."

—British Migraine Association
(as reported in the Florida
Headache Association
newsletter)

"I know this sounds crazy, but if I feel myself getting a migraine, especially with nausea, I try to eat something immediately. Even if food is the last thing in the world I think I want, it sometimes seems to knock the headache right out."

—Jennifer B.

"I tend to get migraines on Saturdays as a letdown after a particularly stressful work week. So when I've had one of those weeks, I'll go into my office on Saturday and sit at my desk for a few minutes to trick myself into thinking I'm working so I won't get a migraine. Believe it or not, it seems to work."

—Misty P.

DON'T BLAME YOURSELF FOR FAILURE

"People think you 'let' the headache take over."

One of the most difficult parts of living with a chronic illness is making peace with the fact that you are not completely in control of your body's responses. Taking as much control as you can will help you feel better about yourself.

If you do everything you can to prevent or remedy a migraine and still wind up with a severe headache, don't be ashamed or feel like you have somehow failed. Even though most people can get some control over their migraines with the right combination of medical care and self-care, no one can control this complex condition one hundred percent of the time.

And even when you slip up in your self-care, you still don't have to feel guilty if you get a migraine. No one expects you to be perfect. Some headaches will occur no matter what you do. You really have no way of knowing for sure whether what you did or did not do had anything to do with your headache. Migraine is an illness—not a punishment.

"Migraine is a legitimate ailment, and that's that."
                    —Nancy Ginn Almond,
                     former newsletter editor,
                     American Council
                     for Headache
                     Education

CHAPTER 17

Menstrual Migraine

Migraine, as we have noted, is considerably more common in women than in men after the age of puberty. The major factor contributing to this difference is the female hormone estrogen. Estrogens, as well as the female hormone progesterone, affect the central nervous system, including the complex systems involving serotonin that play a major role in the development of migraine. (See Chapter 4.)

About 60 percent of women who chart their migraine attacks will note that their headaches are partly or wholly synchronized with the menstrual cycle. For these women the course of their migraine disorder is strongly influenced by hormonal changes throughout life—including menarche, the monthly menstrual cycle, pregnancy, menopause, and the use of synthetic hormones for birth control or for estrogen replacement after hysterectomy or menopause.

TRUE MENSTRUAL MIGRAINE

A woman can be said to have "true menstrual migraine" if her attacks occur during the period two days before, during, and up to three days after her menstrual period and at no other time. Women who also experience attacks at their midcycle, around the time of ovulation, are said to have "menstrually related" migraine.

Women who have headaches during these two critical times of monthly hormonal activity and at other times as well may have a hormonal link to their migraines, but they are not considered to have menstrual migraine.

TREATMENT FOR MENSTRUAL MIGRAINE

True menstrual migraine typically does not respond as well to standard acute and preventive treatments as do other forms of migraine.

One form of treatment that sometimes works for menstrual migraine is the use of ergotamine tartrate as a preventive agent. The drug is given for five to ten days around the time of menstruation, then discontinued for the rest of the month. Women with menstrual migraine rarely have problems with ergot overuse on this regimen, since their headaches are confined to the time around menstruation. Those who can tolerate the drug's side effects often find it very helpful in moderating the severity of their headaches.

Biofeedback is another treatment that helps some women with menstrual migraine. For some women the technique helps when nothing else seems to work. Barb H., for example, had menstrual migraine for twenty years and was completely debilitated by her headaches. After learning biofeedback she was able to moderate her pain enough to return to work.

If women with menstrual migraine do not respond to standard treatments, some physicians will try hormonal treatment with estrogens or with other drugs that affect the hormonal system, including tamoxifen, danazol, and bromocriptine. Such hormonal treatment has not been shown to be consistently helpful, although it is more likely to be effective for women with true menstrual migraine than for women with menstrually related migraine. There is no evidence that hysterectomy is an effective treatment for menstrual migraine.

MENSTRUAL MIGRAINE AND PMS

Many women with migraine who suffer from premenstrual syndrome, or PMS, sometimes believe that their headaches are just another manifestation of that syndrome. Since the timing of PMS and menstrual migraine coincide, this assumption is a logical one, but scientists do not believe it is correct. PMS and menstrual migraine appear to be separate entities, even though both are driven by the woman's hormonal cycle and both affect the central nervous system.

An oblique proof that PMS and menstrual migraine are not the same syndrome is the fact that treatment for PMS usually does not relieve menstrual migraine. Treatment for menstrual migraine usually does not do much to improve PMS either.

PREGNANCY AND MENSTRUAL MIGRAINE

According to some studies, about 60 to 75 percent of women who have migraines will improve during pregnancy, particularly in the second and third trimester. The improvement results because pregnancy tends to stabilize the usual peaks and valleys of estrogen during the monthly cycle. For this reason women who began having menstrual migraine in their teens are more likely to see improvement during pregnancy than women whose migraines are not linked to their menstrual cycle.

Unfortunately the improvement rarely becomes permanent.

Migraines usually begin again in the postpartum period, often in the first few days after the delivery.

In some women who have never had a migraine in their lives, pregnancy, and especially the first trimester, is the start of their migraines. According to a recent review article, about 10 to 15 percent of women who suffer from migraine experienced their first headache during pregnancy.

In one case a clever physician used a woman's first migraine as a clue that she might be pregnant. The twenty-seven-year-old married woman went to her doctor with the typical symptoms of migraine with aura. After making sure she had no neurological problem that would account for the symptoms, the physician made a tentative diagnosis of migraine, and suspecting a hormonal trigger, decided to run a pregnancy test. Sure enough, she was pregnant—and a migraineur.

For a small number of women pregnancy seems to make migraine worse. In a 1990 study researchers found that 7 percent of women with menstrual migraine said their headaches got worse during pregnancy; among women whose migraines were not closely linked to their menstrual cycles, 15 percent said their headaches got worse.

Women who continue to have migraines during pregnancy must give up most of their migraine medications. For headaches that do not respond to nondrug remedies such as heat, cold, biofeedback, or relaxation, acetaminophen with codeine or Demerol can be given under careful supervision.

THE PILL AND MENSTRUAL MIGRAINE

Like pregnancy, the use of oral contraceptives containing estrogen may improve, worsen, or have no effect on a woman's migraines. Women with menstrual migraine may be somewhat more likely to experience headaches when they take oral contraceptives than women whose migraines are not linked to their menstrual cycles.

Some physicians warn all women with migraine, especially those who have migraine with aura, to avoid taking oral contraceptives because they may increase the risk of migraine-related stroke. (See Chapter 20.)

MENOPAUSE, ESTROGEN REPLACEMENT THERAPY, AND MENSTRUAL MIGRAINE

At menopause a woman's natural level of estrogen production falls off sharply. For this reason many women with menstrual migraine experience a reduction in the frequency and severity of their migraine attacks after menopause. While they are going through menopause, however, they may temporarily experience more frequent or more severe attacks as the body copes with fluctuating hormone levels.

The use of synthetic estrogens for estrogen replacement therapy (ERT) has become more widespread now that studies have shown it may help prevent osteoporosis and heart disease. As with the use of birth-control pills, the use of synthetic estrogens during menopause can pose problems for women with menstrual migraine. Some women may see their headaches return, worsen, or become more frequent when they start ERT.

If you want the health benefits of ERT or the relief from menopause symptoms it can provide, your doctor can try several alternatives to taking you off estrogens entirely. One choice would be to change the form of estrogen from the conjugated estrogens commonly prescribed to pure estradiol or estrone. Another possibility is to switch from oral estrogens to a low-dose estrogen patch. The patch maintains a constant level of estrogen in the blood, avoiding the peaks and valleys that appear to contribute to migraine.

Another potentially helpful change would be to switch from cyclical administration of hormones to a noncyclical pattern. Instead of giving estrogen for days one through twenty-five and progesterone on days sixteen through twenty-five, women who are taking ERT after hysterectomy should take a daily dose of estrogen without progesterone. Women who are taking ERT at menopause (without hysterectomy) should take estrogen and progesterone (2.5 mg) daily.

CHAPTER 18

Migraine in Children

Stephanie Z. had experienced severe migraines since childhood. When her fifteen-month-old daughter, Jennifer, began experiencing unexplained bouts of crankiness and crying, Stephanie was sure the problem was migraine.

"I could tell just by the way she acted that the pain was in her head," said Stephanie.

Jennifer's pediatrician was reluctant to treat a toddler for headache but suggested giving her a child's dose of acetaminophen. The medicine sometimes seemed to help.

As Jennifer learned to talk, one of her first sentences was "Head hurt."

Because Stephanie was a longtime migraineur, her diagnosis of her daughter's problem probably was correct. Between 7 and

18 percent of all children experience migraine, and more than half of those who experience adult migraine had their first attacks before they left their teens. More than one million school days are lost to migraine each school year.

Studies have suggested that babies as young as six weeks of age experience migraine attacks. Some researchers believe that head-banging in the crib may be related to migraine pain.

For reasons that are not clear, nearly half of all children with migraine will stop having attacks sometime during their adolescence. Another quarter will stop during their early adult years.

HOW MIGRAINE IN CHILDREN DIFFERS FROM MIGRAINE IN ADULTS

In many respects migraine in children is agonizingly similar to migraine in adults. The pounding head pain, the nausea and vomiting, the aversion to light and sound—all of these can afflict children as well as adults. There are some differences, however, that distinguish migraine in childhood from its adult counterpart.

For reasons that are not clear, children with migraine may experience severe abdominal pain instead of severe headache pain during the "headache" phase of an attack. The abdominal pain, called "abdominal migraine" or "migraine equivalent," may be accompanied by nausea and vomiting and may last for several days. Other migraine equivalents include sudden mood change, dizziness, blurred vision, unexplained fatigue, food cravings, nausea, or loss of appetite.

Since the pain experienced in abdominal migraine mimics many other health problems, your physician will have to rule out other digestive or abdominal problems before making a diagnosis. If your child experiences these symptoms, do *not* assume it is a migraine, even if you have a family history of the disorder.

The symptoms of migraine in children may vary significantly from those found in adults. In particular, aura in children often includes dramatic neurological symptoms such as confusion, hallucinations, dilated pupils, or difficulty speaking. More children than adults experience basilar migraine (see Chapter 5), which may be accompanied by weakness or numbness on both sides of the body, vision problems, temporary balance problems, or dizziness.

SIGNS OF MIGRAINE IN CHILDREN

Because children, especially young children, may not be able to communicate their symptoms, you as a parent will have to observe your child's behavior for warning signs of migraine. Even teens may not always recognize or admit that they're about to have an attack, because they want so much to be "normal."

If you know your child experiences headaches, be alert if he or she suddenly becomes irritable, combative, or withdrawn; mood changes often occur during the preheadache phase of an attack. Since about half of childhood headaches develop when the child wakes up or shortly afterward, be especially alert to crankiness or complaints of discomfort at these times.

Children in the aura phase of migraine may have difficulty speaking or maintaining their balance. They may behave strangely or have trouble focusing their eyes. If you note these signs as the familiar precursors of your child's headaches, have the child lie down in a dark, quiet room and try to relax or sleep. If these symptoms are new to your child, however, or more severe than you have previously noted, call your pediatrician for advice.

TREATING MIGRAINE IN CHILDREN

Some of the medications that work well for adults with migraine can be used for children with migraine. As a general rule, however, physicians are reluctant to prescribe medications as a first resort for children with migraine. Sometimes this reluctance may reflect the doctor's failure to understand how real and painful a migraine is for the child. Most of the time, however, the doctor is concerned about the effects of powerful medications on small bodies and still-developing systems. In addition, medications often have exaggerated side effects in children, because of their smaller size and lower body weight.

For this reason many doctors start by giving children nothing stronger than acetaminophen for pain relief, and by sending them to learn behavioral pain management techniques such as biofeedback and progressive muscle relaxation (see Chapter 15). Recent studies suggest that both techniques work equally well in children with migraine. In some studies as many as half of all children who learned one or both of these techniques were able to reduce the frequency of their headaches and reduce the pain of the headaches that did occur.

Your child is more likely to be successful with these techniques if you are involved and supportive. You will have to help your child maintain the discipline for frequent practice. You will also have to be highly disciplined yourself in cooperating with the objectives of behavioral therapy, by learning to reward your child for using relaxation or biofeedback techniques and trying not to reinforce sickness behaviors. If you can't keep yourself from giving your child some medicine at the first sign of a headache, your child will not be as motivated to try behavioral resources first.

Trigger management is another important part of helping children control their migraines. The same factors that trigger adult migraines can trigger them in children. After every headache you should make it a point to review possible triggers—such as sleep disruption, food items, environmental factors, or unusual stress—to look for patterns. (For a list of possible triggers, see Chapter 6.)

If your child's headaches fail to respond to these nondrug approaches, medication may be necessary. For pain relief acetaminophen usually is the first drug to be tried. For small children it may be administered in suppository or liquid form. If acetaminophen doesn't help the child's head pain, the physician may cautiously try some of the acute medicines used for adult migraine. Never give your child aspirin for a headache. Aspirin has been associated with an uncommon and dangerous disorder called Reye's syndrome, which typically strikes children who have been given aspirin for a viral illness such as the flu.

Like adults, children who have three or more migraine attacks a month usually are candidates for preventive therapy. The same classes of medication that work in adults tend to work in children. Some physicians begin the search for an appropriate preventive agent with a beta blocker like propranolol, but more often the drug cyproheptadine (Periactin) is the first preventive drug used. Periactin does not often help adults, but it can be effective in children. Common side effects are increased appetite and drowsiness.

Another class of drugs that may help children but is not as helpful in adults are the anticonvulsives, particularly phenobarbital and phenytoin (Dilantin).

For many children, as for many adults, sleep is the best answer when a migraine hits. Some children discover this remedy on their own, instinctively going off to a dark, quiet corner and taking a nap. Others may find it hard to sleep because of pain and nausea, or because the very fact of having the attack makes them anxious and restless. Warm or cold compresses sometimes help to soothe the child and reduce the intensity of head pain enough to allow the child to drift off to sleep.

PSYCHOLOGICAL ISSUES IN CHILDHOOD MIGRAINE

Children who have frequent or severe migraines, like children who experience other chronic illnesses, are likely to need special help and support from their parents.

Sick children often personalize their illnesses, viewing illness as a punishment for bad behavior or as a sign that they're different from or not as good as other children. These feelings may cause the child to become withdrawn and isolated, especially if the headaches cause frequent absences from school. As a parent you can help your child by providing frequent reassurance that migraine is a problem that lots of people have. It might help to talk to the child about relatives who have migraine, especially if the child knows and admires these relatives.

Many parents worry that their child may be manipulating them with the illness, seeking special attention and making illness an excuse to avoid chores, school, or other responsibilities in the family. In most cases the child isn't manipulating at all. He or she really hurts, and really can't carry on normal activities during a migraine attack.

If your little migraineur does seem to be looking for some kind of secondary benefit from his or her pain, it isn't a malevolent act. It is only natural for a child to test your limits in this way. The responsibility is yours to help your child understand that sickness is a problem to be dealt with, not a way to get attention or to avoid difficult tasks.

A particularly thorny problem for parents is knowing how much to adapt the family's activities to the child's headaches, especially when there are other children in the family who do not experience headaches. On the one hand parents do not want to make the migraineur feel left out; but on the other hand the migraineur's brothers and sisters may become angry and resentful if everything in the family seems to revolve around one child's headaches.

Communication is a key to preventing these feelings from causing family problems. After several unpleasant scenes when family outings were called off because their middle child had a headache, one couple held a family meeting after dinner to ask their three children what they wanted to do the next time the problem occurred. The children argued angrily for a while about who mom and dad loved more, who was spoiled and who was being *sooo* unfair—then agreed to a perfectly reasonable solution of having their parents take turns staying home with the sick child while the rest of the family went on with the planned activity.

Chronic illness can have a powerful and long-term effect on the entire family. If resentments and anger seem to be getting out of hand in the family, it may help to see a family counselor.

SCHOOL-RELATED PROBLEMS

Headaches during the school year can create difficult problems for students, parents, and teachers. Concerns may range from how to manage a severe headache at school, relate to peers, cope with homework when it hurts to read, and even whether to attend school or not. Fears of failure or falling behind can emerge when headaches become more frequent or severe. Parents may struggle with whether they should push their children or excuse them from activities. Teachers and administrators may question how to respond and what to reasonably expect in school performance.

For headaches severe enough to interfere with functioning, it is crucial that parents, student, health care providers, and school personnel communicate with each other, and agree on a plan for managing severe headaches. The treating physician should provide the school with a clear diagnosis and a practical headache management plan. If medication is required during the school day, the school needs to understand this as well as the limits on frequency of drug use. In turn, parents need to understand the school's medication policy so they can advocate for their child while working within the system. If possible, a quiet location for relaxation and a brief break from class may help keep the child in school and allow a return to the classroom when the pain is under control.

CHAPTER 19

Migraine in Men

"Migraine shouldn't be labeled a 'women's problem.'
Then there would be more money put into resolving it."

Surprisingly little is known about men's unique experience of migraine. Most people—many men included—assume that men don't get "sick headaches" like women do. Ironically a list of famous migraineurs almost always includes far more men than women, among them George Bernard Shaw, Sigmund Freud, Charles Darwin, Thomas Jefferson, and Frédéric Chopin. And even though migraine may be less common among men than among women, it is by no means uncommon among men. An estimated 5.8 million American men have had migraine headaches at some point in their lives.

The true prevalence of migraine among men is hard to discern, because men are more likely to cover up their headaches and less likely to seek medical treatment for headaches than women.

> "My husband and I both get migraines. Our children get headaches, but our two sons refuse to see a doctor about them."

Recent surveys put the ratio of adult female migraineurs to adult male migraineurs at somewhere between three to one and two to one. (See Chapter 3.)

SELF-MISDIAGNOSIS AND SELF-MALTREATMENT

> "I started getting migraines in college. I always thought they were part of a hangover."

> "I remember how irritable my father would get when he had one of his 'sinus' headaches. He'd hold his head and give us frightening looks if the dog barked."

Because men tend to associate migraine with women, they commonly misdiagnose their own experiences of migraine without aura as sinus headaches or as the accompaniment of a hangover. They self-treat the pain with over-the-counter antihistamines or analgesics; occasionally they'll ask the doctor for something stronger, usually an analgesic-codeine combination drug.

Self-treatment, however, can lead to many problems, including rebound headaches and other side-effects from analgesics.

> "I always took care of my headaches myself, with aspirin, until I got a stomach ulcer from taking too much aspirin."

For some men the efforts at self-treatment go to even more dangerous lengths. Several men interviewed for this book admit-

ted that they "borrowed" medication from friends—usually a codeine combination drug or a benzodiazepine tranquilizer like
Valium. Such self-treatment with prescription drugs is risky: these
drugs may have side effects and may not be safe for you. It also is
against the law to use someone else's prescription medication in
this way, particularly abuse-prone drugs like codeine or benzodiazepines.

ARE MEN'S MIGRAINES DIFFERENT?

There is no evidence to show that migraine in men takes any
particular form more often than it does in women. Some British
researchers recently have suggested that there may be some gen-
der-related differences in the triggers for migraine. According to
their survey, men

- are more likely than women to experience "letdown" headaches, particularly on weekends, when they are likely to
  relax, sleep in, and eat later than usual.
- are more vulnerable to work-related stress as a headache
  trigger.

Currently the literature on migraine doesn't contain any evidence that men respond better to certain treatments than women
do. In the field of migraine research the vast majority of studies
involves women patients, in part because the vast majority of
migraine patients who consult doctors (and thus who are available
for studies) are women.

Special Cautions for Men with Migraine

- Don't diagnose your own headaches. If your headaches
  are severe and recurring, talk to your doctor.
- Don't overuse nonprescription medications. Too much,

too often can lead to rebound headaches that worsen the problem.
- Don't self-treat with "borrowed" or illegally obtained prescription drugs.
- Try to keep to your regular schedule on weekends, when you may be more susceptible to letdown headaches.
- Learn about ways to manage stress on the job.
- Don't fall into the trap of male stereotypes:
  - **The Tough Guy:** "It's just a headache. I can take a little pain."
  - **The Grouch:** "Everybody better shut up and leave me alone!"
  - **The Macho Man:** "This isn't some sissy migraine—it's a sinus headache (or hangover headache)."
  - **The Invisible Man:** "Headache? What headache?"

CHAPTER 20

Uncommon Complications of Migraine

As we said at the beginning of this book, migraine is considered a benign disorder because it rarely causes permanent disability or death. In rare cases, however, an unusually severe migraine can lead to serious and sometimes permanent problems.

You will probably never experience the uncommon complications of migraine known as *status migrainosus* and *migraine-related stroke*. But it is important to be aware of them, because they require prompt medical attention if they do occur.

STATUS MIGRAINOSUS

Typically the headache phase of a severe migraine attack lasts less than seventy-two hours. In status migrainosus, however, the attack exceeds this limit, sometimes lasting for a week or more with little or no improvement.

Status migrainosus does not occur very often, but if it happens to you, you should contact your doctor at once or go to an emergency room. Status migrainosus is especially dangerous if you have been experiencing vomiting or diarrhea, because you may become dehydrated. The effects of dehydration can become life threatening if not treated promptly.

People with status migrainosus usually are hospitalized and given intravenous fluids, as well as intravenous drugs to stop the attack and relieve the pain.

MIGRAINE-RELATED STROKE

Even the most severe migraine almost never causes long-term or permanent damage. Migraine-related stroke, also called migrainous infarction or complicated migraine, is an exception. In this infrequent complication of severe migraine, symptoms such as aura, confusion, partial paralysis, or speech impairment persist beyond the duration of the migraine attack. In the uncommon cases where young adults who do not use cocaine or other drugs have a stroke, complicated migraine is often found to be the cause.

Usually the stroke takes place in the posterior or middle cerebral arteries, and very rarely in the brain stem. If it does occur in the brain stem, it usually is associated with basilar migraine, a rare form of migraine characterized by visual impairment on both sides, gait abnormalities, weakness of the limbs, and dizziness.

Researchers don't yet understand how and why migraine causes stroke. For years scientists thought that the stroke was caused by a spasm in the arteries of the brain, just as they used to believe the aura of migraine was caused by arterial spasm (see Chapter 4). When people with migraine have arteriograms done, however, spasm rarely shows up. Now researchers suspect that migrainous stroke may result from the basic neurochemical processes related to migraine.

Since the mechanism of migraine-related stroke is unclear,

scientists aren't sure who is most at risk for having one. Smoking and using oral contraceptives seem to be risk factors. Taking too much ergotamine also increases the risk for migraine-related stroke.

Sometimes the impairments caused by migraine-related stroke improve or disappear with treatment. In other cases they become permanent, as with patients who have strokes caused by other physical problems.

CHAPTER 21

Medication Overuse and Rebound Headaches

"I learned about rebound headaches by reading, not from doctors. Many doctors don't seem to know that some drugs can have rebound effects, or at least they didn't mention it to me."

If you are like many people with migraine, who pop aspirin, acetaminophen, mixed analgesics, or other acute-care medicines every day to get rid of your daily headache, this may be the most important chapter in the book for you. *Your overuse of these drugs may be causing your daily headaches.*

Excessive use of painkillers, ergotamines, and combination drugs are the single most common reason that treatment fails to work for many people with migraine. When these drugs are used on a daily or almost-daily basis, they undermine preventive treatment and actually cause more headaches.

UNDERSTANDING THE REBOUND PHENOMENON

The principle of rebound headaches is easy to understand. If you take a painkiller often, your body gets used to having a certain level of that drug in your bloodstream. If the levels fall below that threshold, you begin to experience the unpleasant effects known as withdrawal symptoms. Among these effects is a diffuse headache that may begin at any place in the head and may eventually cause your whole head to ache.

Many people who are coffee or cola drinkers, for example, know what it is like to get a "caffeine headache" if they miss their morning beverage. The headache is a sign that their blood caffeine levels have fallen below the body's comfort threshold. The same principle is at work in analgesic (painkiller) rebound headache.

Over a period of years the rebounding cycle leads to chronic daily headache—headache that may feel less intense and more diffuse than migraine but that interferes with life as much or more. The process takes place so gradually that you are completely unaware of the connection between your medication use and the headaches you treat with it. You also will continue to have migraine headaches, although you may think of them as merely a more severe variety of the headaches you experience every day.

Rebound Headache Triggers

The following headache drugs are known or suspected to induce rebound headaches if they are taken daily or almost daily (four or more days a week):

Over-the-counter Drugs
- aspirin
- acetaminophen (e.g., Tylenol)
- caffeine (in excess of 500 mg per day—about 3 cups of brewed coffee)

- aspirin and/or acetaminophen with caffeine (e.g., Anacin, Excedrin)

Prescription Drugs
- barbiturate-based combination drugs (e.g., Fiorinal, Fioricet, Esgic)
- narcotic-based combination drugs (e.g., Percocet, Tylox, Vicodin)
- narcotics (e.g., Darvon, Demerol, Dilaudid, morphine)
- ergotamine tartrate (e.g., Cafergot)—should not be used more than one or two days a week, except for prophylactic use around the time of menstruation in women with menstrual migraine

UNDERMINING PREVENTIVE EFFORTS

Another way that overuse of your acute or "rescue" medicines can be harmful is their tendency to interfere with the benefits of your preventive medicines. Preventive medicines work by binding to certain areas of cells, called *receptors*. Scientists think the acute medicines may crowd out the preventive medicines from doing their jobs properly by competing for the biological receptors used by the preventive medicines.

Here's a simple analogy to help explain how that works. Imagine that your house has several holes in the roof, and they leak every time it rains. You've hired someone to replace the roof, but you're worried that your furniture will get wet in the meantime. So every morning, if there's even the tiniest gray cloud in the sky, you grab the ladder and a few shingles and start patching the holes. When the roofers come, they can't work—you have the ladder and the tools!

In certain cases, especially when the rebounding is caused by overuse of opiates such as morphine, the acute medications may make long-term changes in the receptors they bind to. Ironically, the very medicines you count on to help you function from day to day may be keeping you from finding a more effective solution to your headache problem.

SPECIAL DANGERS OF ERGOTAMINE

Ergotamine tartrate, in use to treat migraines since the late 1880s, is derived from a fungus that grows on rye. Used no more than once or twice a week, ergotamine tartrate is a relatively safe and effective drug that helps many people get relief from the pain of migraine. When used more often, however, ergotamine can lead to a number of potentially dangerous problems as well as to rebound headaches.

In excess, ergotamine tartrate may lead to a condition called *ergotism*. Ergotism may lead to mood changes, bizarre behavior, damage to blood vessels, severe muscle cramps, reduction of blood flow to major organs including the brain, epileptic seizures, and stroke. These effects of ergotamine overuse are fairly rare, but they can be extremely serious. If you believe you may be overusing ergotamine medications, report this to your doctor. He or she will help you reduce your dependence on this drug and substitute others that bring relief without the same potential for overuse.

One exception to the general rules about ergotamine use is when ergotamine is prescribed to help prevent menstrual migraine. For this purpose the drug can be taken daily for up to ten days around the menstrual period. It is then discontinued or taken less frequently for the rest of the month.

HOW REBOUND HEADACHES ARE TREATED

If you believe you are overusing any of your analgesics or your ergotamine medications, it is usually not wise to withdraw yourself "cold turkey" from these drugs. If you do, you may find yourself facing several days or even weeks of utter misery from an uncontrollable headache or other unpleasant consequences. Withdrawal from overuse of narcotics or combination drugs can be especially unpleasant and even dangerous if done without medical assistance.

Your physician can help you withdraw gradually and safely from the drugs that are causing you problems. Depending on your degree of dependence, the drugs you are using, and the severity of your headaches, your doctor may withdraw the drugs during a series of outpatient visits or may decide to admit you to the hospital to withdraw the drugs under close medical supervision. If you are admitted to the hospital, he or she may give you DHE intravenously, along with an antinausea drug, to help prevent headaches during withdrawal. If necessary you will be given other pain medications, such as nonsteroidal antiinflammatory drugs (NSAIDs), as your troublesome analgesics are tapered off.

After you have begun withdrawing from the drugs, you may experience a "washout period" during which you will be intensely sensitive to pain and may experience more headache pain than usual. This period usually lasts no more than a month.

According to researchers about half of patients who are carefully withdrawn from rebound-inducing drugs experience a 50 percent reduction in the intensity and frequency of their headaches within a month; within three months, four out of five patients experience similar improvement. The treatment does not end your migraines, but it can free you from the daily headaches that characterize the rebound cycle. With these headaches out of the way your doctor can then concentrate on finding appropriate and effective acute and preventive medications for your migraines.

CHAPTER 22

When Treatment Doesn't Seem to Help

Headache specialists estimate that at least 85 to 90 percent of people with migraine can find significant relief with currently available treatments. If you are a migraineur who hasn't found a satisfactory treatment, you may read a statistic like that and see it as proof that the experts are out of touch with the reality of living with migraine. Or you may believe it proves that the physician's definition of "success" may not feel much like success to you.

A surprisingly large number of migraineurs believe that nothing can be done to help them, or that they've "tried it all" and failed to get any control over their headaches. There are many reasons why treatment doesn't help some people at some times. But in many of these cases you may not necessarily be as powerless as you may feel. Often there is something you can do to improve the chances that treatment will work for you.

If treatment hasn't worked for you so far, see if your situation matches any of the barriers to treatment success described in this chapter. Then try again!

POSSIBLE BARRIERS TO TREATMENT SUCCESS

You Have Not Consulted a Doctor

Many people with migraine believe they can't get help for their headaches—*without ever asking for help.* If you have severe headaches that do not respond to over-the-counter medications, or that have been increasing in frequency, see your doctor.

You Haven't Found the Right Help

If your doctor dismissed your headaches or prescribed just a painkiller that you've been taking four or more days a week, you need to see another doctor, preferably one who specializes in headache. (See Chapter 9.)

Medications Make You Feel Too Bad

Migraine medications are powerful and often have side effects. Part of the process of selecting a treatment is finding a drug you can live with, one whose side effects are less unpleasant and troublesome for you than the headache. If a drug has side effects you can't tolerate, *don't give up on the treatment process.* Let your doctor try another drug or another treatment plan. Too many people give up too soon and miss out on the opportunity to find relief.

You Are Not Taking Medication Properly

Taking preventive and acute medications on the right schedule and in the right dosage is essential for success in treating migraine. If you are not following your treatment plan for any reason, talk to your doctor. He or she can help you understand how to follow your medication schedule or may prescribe something else that you are able to take as directed.

You Are Taking Too Many Painkillers

When ergotamines, over-the-counter and prescription painkillers, or combination drugs are used more than three times a week, they can lead to intractable headaches that eventually occur every day. (See Chapter 21.)

You Smoke or Are Frequently Around Secondhand Smoke

Smoking interferes with the effectiveness of certain medicines used to treat migraine. Cigarette smoke also is a frequent migraine trigger. Quitting smoking—or spending less time in smoke-filled environments—may greatly improve the success of your migraine treatment.

TRUE INTRACTABLE MIGRAINE

At any given time a small number of people who have none of these barriers to successful treatment will experience what is called *true intractable migraine* or *chronic intractable migraine.* These are people who have received the best available treatments and who try their best to manage their lifestyle and their triggers, but do not receive significant or sustained relief.

Scientists do not know why some people fail treatments that help millions, or why some people may fail all treatments for a short time and later find relief. This same phenomenon occurs in the case of other chronic illnesses such as asthma or diabetes. Sometimes the treatments simply don't work, or work for a while and then stop working. Other times the side effects of treatment are too severe.

If you are one of the few people who currently experience

intractable migraine, don't lose heart. Rarely is someone doomed to have intractable migraine forever. Sometimes the period during which their headaches are out of control lasts a few months. For a very few unlucky people the situation may persist for years. Keep working with your headache specialist, who will monitor new treatments and new ways to administer current treatments.

CHAPTER 23

The Future of Migraine Treatment

The 1990s saw a virtual explosion of knowledge regarding the biological basis of migraine. Fortunately for migraine sufferers, this scientific knowledge led to the emergence of a new class of drugs that has transformed the acute treatment of migraine.

In 1991, sumatriptan (Imitrex) became the first drug in this new class of specific migraine medications, ushering in the "triptan era." In the late 1990s, the Food and Drug Administration (FDA) approved three additional triptans: zolmitriptan (Zomig), naratriptan (Amerge), and rizatriptan (Maxalt) for the acute treatment of migraine. As this edition goes to press, several others, including eletriptan (Relpax), frovatriptan, and almotriptan, are in final development or approval stages. (Contact your physician or the American Council for Headache Education for the latest information on their status.)

The obvious question to ask is: Why do we need several drugs from the same class with the same mechanism of action? Researchers speculated that patients could receive quicker, more consistent, and lasting pain relief if new compounds could be developed that were more rapidly and consistently absorbed, that penetrated the barrier separating the blood from the brain, and that lasted longer in the bloodstream.

Based upon these goals, the race to develop the "ultimate" triptan began. Drug companies vie for the triptan that possesses one or more attributes (rapid onset, consistent relief, tolerability, low recurrence) that make it distinct and unique among the competition in this class of medications.

Without question, the clear victor in the "war of the triptans" is the migraine patient, for in their effort to develop the ultimate triptan, the pharmaceutical industry provides patients and physicians with a formidable arsenal with many options for migraine relief.

But triptans aren't the only weapons to consider in the ongoing battle against migraine. Dozens of other drugs are being studied for use in migraine treatment, including new preventive medications. Exciting genetic research in this field is also underway.

The future of migraine treatment is very promising.

PART THREE

Living
with
Migraine

CHAPTER 24

Coping with Emotions

"There are times when I feel angry, sad, and depressed. I feel totally out of control and wonder if I've done something wrong. The helplessness and frustration of knowing I'm going to lose a day or more of my life to a migraine can be overwhelming. That's especially true when I'm surrounded by people who say, 'Oh, you have *another* headache.' "

"I have been fearful of what people thought about me—that I was lazy, seeking attention, or avoiding going back to work. I even wondered what my husband thought."

The illness of migraine has powerful effects on the migraineur's life that reach far beyond the actual hours of pain. People who experience migraine find themselves at the mercy of a recurrent, invisible illness that may resist treatment, flare unpredictably at the most inconvenient times even if it is being successfully treated, and leave others wondering how anything with no outward sign can be *that* painful.

These experiences stir up powerful emotions that whirl through the migraineur's life, even when no headache is present. Some of these emotions include

- **Powerlessness.** You can't predict when a migraine attack will come. You can't always prevent them by medication, trigger-management techniques, or relaxation. Your rescue medicine may not stop one on the way.
- **Guilt.** You are convinced you're not "pulling your weight" on the job or in your family. You feel like you are letting your spouse, partner, kids, co-workers down. You believe you bring the headaches on yourself by not being careful enough about triggers.
- **Shame.** You believe your headaches are a sign that you can't handle pressure as well as other people. You sense others' judgment of you, and you think they are probably right.
- **Depression.** Even the headache-free times seem to lose their attractiveness. You can't get interested in anything, even your favorite pursuits.
- **Anger.** You think, *Why me?* as the headache comes on. You can't understand why your family doesn't cooperate more when you have a headache.
- **Isolation.** You sense others' lack of understanding about migraine. You feel that no one, not even your family, can truly comprehend your pain. You feel that others are not as sympathetic as they might be.
- **Regret.** You realize how much of your life has been spent in darkened rooms. You wonder what your life would have been like up to now if you didn't have migraines.

Don't feel ashamed if these emotions get the better of you from time to time. As a person with a chronic illness your life is very complicated.

A positive way to cope during difficult times is to make a commitment to finding help. Some people look to a support group; others find a compassionate and understanding therapist or counselor. The one thing you should *not* do is to resign yourself to unhappiness.

Steps on the Path to Emotional Health

- Acknowledge your feelings and find appropriate ways to express them without attacking others.
- Ask for what you want from others. Don't expect the people who love you to know what you need without your telling them. Be as specific as possible, but realize they also have a right to refuse.
- Learn to say a guilt-free, unapologetic no when others make demands while you have a migraine or sense one coming on. You can say it in a loving tone, but learning to meet your body's need for rest and quiet is a priority.
- Don't feel required to be cheerful. That's not to say migraine is an excuse to be unkind, grouchy, or insensitive. It does mean acknowledging that feelings of frustration, anger, and resentment are perfectly normal responses to chronic pain. Once you have acknowledged the presence and reality of your feelings, you are in a better position to cope with the situation.
- Treat yourself with love and respect, and others will follow in kind.
- Treat those around you with love and respect.
- Don't go through it all alone. Find yourself a network of support: a headache- or chronic-pain support group, a therapist who understands migraine, a religious counselor, or sympathetic friends.

STARTING A SUPPORT GROUP

"I wish there were more support groups. I feel sorry for
my friend who doesn't have one."

"My support group helps a lot. It's good to be able to
speak out about migraine and to know there are people
there who understand. We swap therapies and ideas."

The emotional storms that accompany chronic illness often
can be greatly diminished by finding or starting a support group.
Support groups provide a feeling of family for people with similar
experiences.

Meeting regularly with people who know exactly what you
mean when you say, "I felt guilty when I had to leave my family to
lie down in a dark room," can help you feel less alone. Strangers
soon become good friends because of your shared experiences.
Through listening and sharing with others who have faced the
same challenges, you learn techniques and coping mechanisms to
add to your own repertoire of coping strategies.

If you've never attended support-group meetings, you may be
apprehensive about telling your life story to total strangers. Don't
worry—there's no rule that requires you to say a word. If you are
shy, you can take comfort in knowing that most groups have a
designated facilitator for the meeting, part of whose job it is to
help newcomers feel welcomed and comfortable.

As someone who probably has experienced criticism for your
headache-related behavior, you will be glad to know that members of support groups make a special effort to be nonjudgmental.
They work together to provide a space for each other that is safe
and free of criticism.

Support groups typically include anywhere from three to ten
people. They meet in individuals' homes, churches, synagogues,
libraries, community centers, or anywhere in your community that
offers meeting rooms. Many groups choose someone to lead the
meeting. Sometimes a group has a permanent leader, or they may

rotate leadership each month. The leader's responsibility is to make sure that no one feels judged harshly and that everyone who wants to participate in the discussion has an opportunity.

Occasionally support groups will have guest speakers come in to provide information about new treatments or medications for headaches or simply to provide encouraging personal stories about migraine management. The group also may become involved in other projects together, such as talking to local emergency-room personnel about the needs of migraine patients.

The critical component of a support group is that group members learn to participate in the management of their migraine, not passively accept migraine as their lot in life. Group members learn from each other. A great testament to the importance of support groups in members' lives is that many will come even if they are having a headache!

Tips for Starting a Support Group

- Link up with existing networks of support groups to benefit from their experience. (For information about these networks, see the "Resources" section at the end of this book.)
- Put up notices in your public library or other community locations asking people to call if they're interested.
- If there is a headache clinic or chronic-pain treatment program in your area, contact someone there and ask them to publicize your meeting.
- Set up an initial organizational meeting.
- Pass out a questionnaire at the first meeting asking people when they would prefer to meet, how often, and where. Be sure to get names, addresses, and phone numbers.
- Decide on a format for the group. Will the group be open to new members, or closed after a certain period of time? Will one person be the leader? Will leadership/facilitation rotate through the membership? Will

you invite experts to speak? Will you invite people with
migraine to speak? Will there be a question-and-answer
period following the speaker? Will the group be basi-
cally an information-sharing and support group for
each other, or is outreach an important goal for you?
- Establish a time and place for another meeting and
agree on ways to publicize the meeting to others.

GETTING PROFESSIONAL HELP
FROM A THERAPIST

"I started out thinking that therapy was just talk, talk,
talk. I was very wrong. I've really learned a lot about
what to do when I feel chaotic and helpless. My therapist didn't know a thing about migraine when we started
—but she does now."

"Family therapy would help everyone learn to deal with
migraine."

Psychotherapy is no longer considered just for people with
mental illnesses. For many ordinary people psychotherapy is a
way to learn new methods of coping with the challenges of life.

Psychotherapy can be helpful during times when you are trying to manage the emotions caused by life with migraine. If there
are underlying psychological issues, they can be addressed in the
therapeutic setting as well.

Some people avoid therapy because they are afraid it will
involve years of weekly visits and thousands of dollars. Today,
however, short-term psychotherapy lasting a few months is very
common and can be quite effective.

Shop wisely for a therapist. Get recommendations from
friends and family. If there is a headache clinic or chronic-pain
treatment program in your area, find out whether they have a list
of psychotherapists knowledgeable about those problems. Be sure

to interview several by telephone or in person before making a decision. A short telephone interview may help you determine if you have rapport with the therapist and would be comfortable working with him or her. The therapist you choose should be knowledgeable about migraine and understand that headaches are not "caused" by a psychological problem.

You don't have to wait until you are in extreme circumstances before you go to a therapist for help. But if you are having extreme feelings, *do not delay.* It is especially important to seek help from a professional counselor or therapist if

- you find yourself entertaining thoughts of suicide between headaches.
- you lose interest in things you've always enjoyed doing, even when you are not having headaches.
- you begin avoiding going out of the house, avoiding going places where you've had migraines before, or if you're often thinking morbid thoughts that your migraines are an ominous sign that you may die suddenly. Although not wanting to get a migraine or having some fear of being somewhere and getting a migraine is perfectly normal, avoidance behavior is a sign that you are in deep distress. You can receive help to deal with your fears.

Interview Questions for Therapists or Counselors

When seeking a counselor or therapist, it's important to find someone who has an accurate understanding of migraine or who is open to learning from you. When you are interviewing therapists, try asking the following questions:

- **Have you worked with clients with migraine or chronic pain?**
  If the therapist responds with success stories of people cured by dealing with underlying psychological issues, beware. If the therapist says he or she has worked with

clients with migraine and that there are ways to learn to feel more in control of your life, then you're on the right track.

- **Would you be open to reading some materials on migraine?**
  Any good therapist will indicate an openness and willingness to learn. If the therapist seems to think he or she already knows it all, call someone else.

- **What is your idea about the relationship between stress and migraine?**
  If the therapist seems to think stress causes migraine, you could be in trouble. If the therapist says that stress can be a contributing factor to migraine for some people, you may well have a winner.

- **Do you believe that people can cure themselves of migraine?**
  If the therapist answers yes, it's time to call another therapist.

Remember, a therapist doesn't necessarily have to be headache-prone to be able to help you. He or she simply needs to view migraine as an illness that affects your emotions and complicates your life, not as a sign that you have emotional problems.

TAPPING YOUR MOST IMPORTANT RESOURCE

"When we're pain free, we're really happy, upbeat people."

Therapists and support groups can be vital resources as you struggle to keep your emotional balance despite migraine. But let's not ignore the most important resource of all: your own inner strength. It takes tremendous courage and inner strength to face recurrent bouts of excruciating pain and the disruption that results from migraine. You need to give yourself credit for that strength.

Despite years of frustration, ineffective treatments, dashed hopes, humiliation, and excruciating pain, you *carry on.* You find or make ways to live your life, to do your job, to parent your children, to make a home for yourself or your family. Even when your migraines are bad, and you can't do all that you might want to do, you do what you can. Very few migraineurs give up on life.

Your successes are an incredible testament to the power of the human spirit. Be proud of what you have been able to do in your life despite carrying an enormous burden. Don't demean your achievements by wondering what you might have done or could have been. Appreciate what you are: a person who takes one of life's sourest lemons—chronic, recurrent pain—and makes lemonade.

Don't think of yourself as a migraine *sufferer.* Celebrate yourself as a migraine *survivor.*

CHAPTER 25

Migraine and Family Life

"Everything about migraine is hard on my family. My changing jobs so often has been hard on us. Finances have been hard—we get ahead, and then we go in a hole."

For many migraineurs the most painful experiences surrounding migraine come from its effects on the quality of family life. Every time a family outing must be canceled or a family member left behind to cope with a headache alone, everyone in the family experiences a mixed bag of anger, guilt, frustration, and sense of loss. Many migraineurs feel terribly guilty about their children, who lose access to a parent every time the headache strikes and who may worry excessively about Mommy's or Daddy's health.

Between the grown-ups in the household migraine causes many practical problems with everything from child care to finances. In addition the problems that happen in any relationship, from sex to money to in-laws to division of responsibility, become supercharged with emotion. The strain of coping with chronic illness stresses some marriages to the breaking point.

As difficult and painful as family life may become when your migraines are at their worst, it is by no means inevitable that migraine will end your marriage or deprive your children of their childhood. For many families the process of learning to cope with chronic illness provides an opportunity for tremendous growth. What usually makes the difference is a sense of common purpose: that migraine is not just "Mom's problem" or "Junior's problem" but *everyone's* problem.

This chapter is addressed to you, the person experiencing migraine. Chapter 26, "Living with a Migraineur," is addressed to the people who live with you.

THE DYNAMICS OF MIGRAINE

A family is a complex web of relationships: strong and flexible, but very much interrelated. Your headaches are a family affair, like any other challenge that faces a member of the family.

Migraine can disrupt a family's pattern of relating in several ways.

- **The stresses caused by migraine may make existing problems worse, adding additional strain to the family.** For example, if a husband and wife are having financial problems, the cost of migraine treatment may add to the burden and make them more anxious.
- **Migraine may become the "scapegoat," taking the blame for other problems in the family.** For example, if a couple are having problems disciplining their teenagers, they may blame the problems on migraine: "If you weren't always shut away with a headache, the kids would know what's expected of them." "If you spent more time with the chil-

dren, they would at least have one parent to count on when I'm down with a headache."

- **Migraine may expose underlying communication problems that make it difficult for the family to cope with adversity.** For example, a couple who never learned how to express anger without becoming explosive or manipulative may not have a clue about where to begin talking about the frustrations of migraine.

In many respects migraine becomes a litmus test for the family's overall emotional development. A family in which problems routinely are discussed and solutions worked out will have distinct advantages in coping with migraine.

FEELING ALONE

"My father felt guilty because he has migraine, and my husband doesn't understand. We have no communication about headache."

"My husband and his family deny my migraines. I have no support from my husband."

"My husband is irritated that I have migraine."

From the point of view of a person who gets migraines, perhaps the most painful feeling is of being on the outside within one's own family. Migraineurs routinely report that their families either don't believe the extent of their pain or else believe they brought it on themselves by something they did voluntarily.

MIGRAINE AND SEXUAL INTIMACY

"Not tonight, I have a headache" may be one of the most damaging jokes ever made at migraineurs' expense. And there may be a bitter irony involved: some research has suggested that migraineurs may experience intense sexual arousal during some phase of their migraine attack, probably as a result of serotonin disturbances.

Ironies aside, migraine often does have a profound effect on sexual intimacy. Frequent attacks leave little time for nurturing a sexual relationship. Some medications may depress sexual interest or interfere with male potency. Even more insidious, the anger and resentment built up by partners who feel abandoned, misunderstood, or overburdened may play themselves out in the bedroom. One partner may withhold sex out of anger, while the other increasingly demands sexual attention as a demonstration of the partner's love or as a duty of marriage.

A loss of sexual intimacy does not have to accompany migraine. If the problem is interest or potency, talk to your physician. He or she may consider changing your medication or dosage, or may ask you to consult with a psychiatrist or psychologist to be evaluated for depression. Similarly, if your headache treatments are not controlling your migraines enough for you to carry on your personal life, you may need a medication change.

If your problems are a result of taking negative emotions to bed with you, you may need the help of a counselor or family therapist to help you learn more constructive ways to handle anger and resentment. Don't let the problem fester too long: the trust and intimacy found in sexual relations can help you and your partner through many difficult times with your headaches.

MIGRAINE AND THE FAMILY BUDGET

Sex and money vie for top honors as the number one source of marital discord. Migraine brings with it many financial stresses that can add to existing financial problems. The cost of medical care, medications, and medical insurance may run to thousands of dollars each year. Lost wages caused by excessive absenteeism or job loss add to the burden, as does the cost of child care and other special services needed to take up the slack in a family with children when one parent is incapacitated.

Money is an emotional subject for nearly all of us. Financial worries call up fears of privation and humiliation that may or may not be rational. If partners did not have an understanding about financial priorities before migraine complicated the picture, they may find themselves at odds about whom to pay first with the money they have.

The first step in coping with financial issues is getting a true picture of where you are. Sometimes you will be able to identify the key financial issues easily: for example, poor health-insurance coverage, or unstable income, or a need to budget more effectively. If your situation is complicated or desperate, however, you may need the help of a credit counselor or financial planner or of someone in the social services department of your city or county.

The key to living with the financial demands of migraine, however, rests with you and your family. Once all of you truly accept the fact that migraine is an illness, and is not anyone's fault, you may be better able to cope with its financial effects. Many times worry about money disguises a greater concern about the future: *What will happen in a few years? Will Mom (or Dad) get better—or worse? Will there be money for me to meet my basic needs?* If such basic concerns can be given voice through patient, honest communication sessions, greater understanding can often be reached.

MIGRAINE AND PARENTING

The most painful emotions surrounding migraine often come from conflicts with children or conflicts between parents over children. In some cases the problems may result directly from migraine. You may not be able to pick the kids up at school consistently, for example, or you may miss important parent-child activities because of your headaches. These problems may lead to intense conflicts with your spouse, who may not be able to pick up the slack easily if he or she is working.

If your child also is headache-prone, you may experience intense guilt over having passed the tendency on. Your guilt may lead you to overextend yourself when the child is ill, taking all the care chores on yourself, disrupting your sleep and thereby risking your own health.

The most poignant feelings, however, come when you realize how dramatically your children's lives are altered by your migraines.

"Whenever we were ready to do something special, it seemed that my mother would have a headache. In my child's mind she was a mean mommy who just didn't want to do things."

You also may recognize your children's fears that you will die or be permanently incapacitated by one of your attacks.

These feelings may be especially difficult to handle if you and your spouse have differences of opinion about child-rearing or if you and your spouse have other, serious unresolved problems. As with sex and money, children become a way to fight by proxy about all the basic issues in your relationship.

For starters, let up on any guilt you may feel about "stealing your children's childhood." There's little evidence to show that having a parent with migraine does permanent damage to a child's potential or growth. Then try to talk honestly and openly with your spouse or your children about practical problems, such as picking the kids up after school. Start with small problems, and look for workable solutions. When you have experienced successes with these smaller issues, you can build on those successes to approach the more complex questions related to your migraines.

THE LOADED ISSUE OF "SECONDARY GAIN"

"I believed my mother controlled us with her headaches. Recently my forty-five-year-old daughter told me she felt the same way about me!"

If any one accusation comes up more frequently than any other in arguments between a headache-prone person and his or her spouse, it is the plaintive wail, "You manage to do the things *you* want to do, but you always get a migraine when it's time for you to do something for me."

No statement hurts a migraineur more, because it implies that the migraineur somehow *chose* to have a migraine attack as a way of manipulating the family. Anyone who has ever had a migraine attack knows that to be a hopelessly false assumption. Most migraineurs would sooner cut off a leg than will a migraine on themselves.

Yet there may be a bitter crumb of truth that migraineurs derive some "secondary gain" at the time they have a migraine. Even though migraine has a biological cause, the person with the migraine may also receive some "benefits" from his or her suffering. Although no one would choose to have excruciating pain in order to get out of going to school, washing the dishes, or attending a class reunion, those benefits may accrue to the person with the migraine. The person may or may not seek out those benefits whenever he or she gets a migraine.

Secondary gain may be one reason why family members feel controlled by the person with the migraine. If a wife has gotten a headache every time her husband wanted her to go fishing with him, does that mean that his wife is consciously setting out to get a migraine on these occasions, or is somehow exaggerating the pain? Of course not. It does mean that she may be unconsciously using her migraine attacks for secondary gain.

Another example of secondary gain at work is the child who has a severe migraine at school. The fear and embarrassment associated with having the headache and vomiting may be so overwhelmingly embarrassing that the child doesn't want to go back to school. When the child is forced to go back, he or she becomes so anxious that another migraine is triggered. The cycle keeps repeating itself, and each time the child gets to stay home from school for a day or so. The child truly is suffering from the headache, but the secondary gain is that he or she doesn't have to go to school.

The acknowledgment that some migraineurs experience secondary gain should not be taken as "blaming the victim." Instead, it highlights the importance of open, honest communication in the family. Although the family members are not right in thinking that the migraineur really causes the headache, they may be pointing out a benefit that the migraineur may not be consciously seeking or acknowledging.

If there is any grain of truth to your family members' citing of secondary gain, don't waste time feeling guilty. You need to take steps to reduce the pressures on your life and to find ways to ask for what you need directly.

YOUR BUILT-IN SUPPORT GROUP

In discussing all the stresses on family life caused by migraine, it's important not to overlook the tremendous emotional support many migraineurs receive from their families.

Because migraine often runs in families, many people say that fellow headache-prone family members are their most accessible and helpful support group.

> "My father has been a big help. He has migraines, and just having him to talk to, to know I wasn't going crazy and I wasn't abnormal, was great."

A spouse who experiences other types of headache than migraine also can be a source of support.

"I have the most understanding husband. He has cluster headaches, so he can identify. He's incredibly sympathetic, and I know I couldn't have made it without that."

Sometimes even non–headache-prone family members can empathize and be supportive.

"I'm lucky. My whole family is supportive. My husband changes the ice pack in the night. It's embarrassing he's so kind."

If you are not now fortunate enough to have a supportive family, don't despair. Family life is a process. The family is a place where people can learn to grow.

The key to this learning is open, honest dialogue. Many times you will find that your family's apparent lack of sympathy masks other emotions. Breaking the emotional silence and unmasking the hidden feelings may show all of you new ways to relate and to help each other cope with a sad situation that isn't anybody's fault.

Sometimes family counseling or participation in family support groups can be valuable tools to get everyone talking to each other. As in other chronic illnesses family members often find they need support, a place to vent their feelings, and some advice on how to cope constructively.

"Mom used to be in denial. Now she's a member of ACHE."

"We hardly talked about the effect that my headaches were having on the family—until things bottomed out. The family was hurting, they truly wanted to know more so that they would not feel helpless and uninvolved."

Finding healing for the family is not dependent on curing your migraines. It is dependent on working together as a family to understand migraine as a chronic disabling condition, to learn to communicate openly, and to remain as flexible as possible.

Migraineurs: Key Facts to Remember About Migraine's Effects on Family Life

- Migraine rarely is the cause of family problems. Most often it just makes existing problems obvious, or makes them worse.
- Your family—especially your children—probably feel frightened and helpless when you have a headache. Sometimes they may hide their concern, perhaps even by seeming not to care at all. Don't be fooled. Be sure to help your family understand what migraine is and is not.
- The whole family, including you, need positive ways to vent the anger they feel at your headaches. Make time for this release of pent-up anger during your headache-free time.
- If a family member accuses you of wanting to get out of chores or avoid family activities by using your migraines as a convenient excuse, try not to react defensively.
  - First you need to make sure your family member understands that you do not cause your headaches and that they are very real.
  - Second (and this is the hard one), you need to ask yourself if there is any grain of truth to the person's statement. If there is, you need to take steps to reduce the pressures on your life and to find ways to ask for what you need directly. Open communication is essential in a family affected by migraine.
- Your family is not alone is being disrupted by migraine. Every family with a migraineur faces the same issues. You may find great comfort in attending a headache support group.
- Get help if your family can't resolve migraine-related

problems. See a family therapist who is experienced in dealing with people in chronic pain. And go before problems become critical—don't wait until your family has collapsed under the strain.

CHAPTER 26

Living with a Migraineur: Special Advice for Family Members

"I'm worried about Mommy being sick."
—Alex R., 4½ years old

The challenge of illness always is difficult for a family to bear. How much more difficult when the illness is migraine—unpredictable, easily misunderstood, devastatingly painful, and complex to treat.

If you are the spouse, partner, child, or parent of a migraineur, your life is nearly as much affected by the illness as that of your family member. When the migraineur is suffering, you suffer too. When the migraineur can't sustain normal activities, you may wind up with more responsibility than would be fair under ordinary circumstances. When the migraineur can't go out, you may find your pleasures curtailed too—or you may feel guilty for going on alone.

As a family member of a migraineur it is important that you recognize that yours is a difficult situation.

A MIX OF EMOTIONS

"I worry a lot—mostly about her driving when the aura comes on and possibly having an accident."

"I feel guilty sometimes, because I passed this on to my daughter."

As the family member of a migraineur, you may find yourself prey to a host of painful emotions. Some of the most common ones are anger, guilt, frustration and fear.

Anger: Powerful, irrational anger at the headaches is a very common feeling among family members of migraineurs. The problem is, your loved one may mistake your anger at the headache for anger at her or him, resulting in hurt feelings and guilt for both of you. Sometimes your anger may, in fact, be anger at your loved one—because he or she isn't feeling well, because nothing seems to help, because you are stuck with more responsibility than you want. Even if you know the anger isn't justified, it may just be there anyway.

Guilt: Sometimes you may feel what is called "survivor guilt": "Why am I fine, when someone I love so much is hurting so badly?" Other times your guilt may stem from a mistaken sense of responsibility: "If I could just do enough or just do the right thing, the pain would go away." You also may feel guilty for feeling angry at someone you know is ill.

Frustration: You may feel frustrated if you and your loved one keep doing everything "right" but see no change in the headache pattern. This frustration may express itself in many ways, such as insisting that your loved one change doctors, making hostile phone calls to your loved one's unsympathetic boss, picking on your kids for small infractions, or even blowing up at your loved one and suggesting that he or she "could" get better, but won't.

Fear: Like your loved one you may worry that the headaches are a sign of some terrible illness: a brain tumor, for example, or an impending stroke.

Learning to recognize these emotions in yourself is an important first step. The next step is to understand that all of them are just feelings, and it's perfectly okay to feel them sometimes. But you need to recognize that you don't have to let these emotions rule you when you interact with your loved one during a headache crisis. If you're angry or disappointed, fearful or frustrated, acknowledge it to yourself, but don't act it out with the person with the migraine.

THE BEST WAYS TO HELP

Over and over migraineurs say that what they need most from you as a family member is a sense of being believed, understood, and cared about. The sense of isolation that accompanies chronic pain is hard for migraineurs to bear. Because migraineurs also feel a sense of guilt for "spoiling everything," they also fear the family's rejection.

A simple expression of love, sympathy, and a desire to help makes your loved one feel less alone and less guilty. That moment of connection can be a powerful bond between you, despite the isolating force of the illness.

Another good way to be supportive is to help the person take charge of his or her pain. Migraineurs often feel that their headaches control their lives. Part of their task in learning to treat their headaches is to learn how to have some measure of control, if not over when the headaches come, then at least over how they respond to the pain.

There's a fine line between helping someone take charge and taking charge for them. For example, if the person with the headache asks for a cold cloth or for you to take the kids into another room, these small kindnesses may help a great deal. Asking you to do these things may be part of your loved one's regaining a sense of control over the immediate circumstances of the headache.

If you offer to help, do so in a specific, concrete way. "May I bring you an ice pack?" "May I massage your head?" But if you call the doctor before your husband asks, if you scoop up your wife and take her to the emergency room, if you bring your teenage daughter her medicine and demand she take it, or if you do anything else that puts you in charge of the headache, you may be reinforcing your loved one's sense of helplessness. Instead of bettering the situation, you may be preventing the person from following his or her own sense of what to do to control the headache.

If you find that you can't break the habit of taking charge, or if you find that your loved one can't get used to your not taking charge when the headache sets in, it may be time to get some family counseling. You may need a trained professional to help you and your loved one learn to disentangle love from dependency and learn to give and take only what's helpful. It is a good idea to find a counselor experienced in dealing with people who have headache, or at least with those who have chronic pain. If your doctor can't suggest anyone, find out whether your local hospital has a headache treatment program or a chronic pain treatment program. Often a psychologist or family counselor will be a consultant to these programs, and he or she will be familiar with the issues your family faces.

TAKING CARE OF YOURSELF

"It's very, very stressful for my husband and me. My daughter, who is thirty-nine, has gotten migraine headaches every three weeks since puberty. They last for several days. When she has them, she can't get out of bed, can't cook, can't function, can't do anything. She can't work full time. We help support her. We take care of her, but she doesn't live with us—it's a matter of pride to her. I don't know what's going to happen to her when we're gone. That hangs over us all the time."

Living with someone who has a chronic illness is taxing on the mind, body, and spirit. You will feel at the end of your resources sometimes. That feeling is perfectly normal. It is not a sign that you don't love your spouse or child. It is not a sign that you're a selfish, inconsiderate lout. It is just a sign that you are human.

The best action you can take if you begin to feel burned-out is to get a respite. After you have done what you can to help the person with the migraine, do something nice for yourself. Treat yourself to a night out with friends. If there are children in the family, play a game with them, or take them for a walk or a movie.

It's perfectly okay to play hookey for an hour, a day, or a weekend. To make yourself and your migraineur feel more secure, you can set up a plan for what to do in case a bad headache hits. If a trip to the emergency room is necessary, how will your loved one get there and back? If he or she can't handle the kids, who can come and take care of them?

It may be painful to you to tell your loved one that you need some time off. It may call up hostility from the migraineur: after all, he or she can't take time off from being headache-prone. Airing these feelings openly and honestly, however, may bring everyone closer. If you are at all worried, you may want to talk to someone you trust—a therapist, religious counselor, family friend, or support-group member—before you broach the subject.

An important preventative against burnout is to remember that you are not responsible for curing your loved one's pain. You *can't* cure it. In fact, you can do very little at all beyond being understanding and showing your compassion in small kindnesses. That fact may be a source of anguish, but it also can be very liberating.

To help you keep your perspective, especially when the migraines are frequent and the day-to-day demands great, you may benefit from taking part in headache support groups, especially ones that are organized for family members. The group members may help you to see that you are not alone, that your feelings of helplessness, frustration, guilt, and anger are perfectly normal responses to a stressful situation.

THE ULTIMATE GOAL: A PARTNERSHIP OF HOPE

Treatment for a chronic illness like migraine is a lifelong process. Coming to accept that may be hard for you and for the migraineur in your family. We all want to believe that medicine can fix anything—but migraine isn't fixable. It is, however, highly treatable under the right circumstances.

In your family you can create the right circumstances for successful treatment by encouraging communication. Talk about your feelings, your needs, and your hopes. Encourage your loved one to do the same, and *really* listen.

Ultimately, you and your loved one must learn to accept headaches (or at least the possibility of headaches) as part of your life, a challenge to be met like other challenges facing your family. With good communications you and your family member can join together in a partnership of hope, mutually committed to seeing that everyone in your family has the best possible quality of life.

**Family Members: Key Facts to Remember
When Migraine Disrupts Your Life**

- Your loved one doesn't cause the headaches. They are part of a biological disorder.
- Migraine may disrupt your life or spoil your plans from time to time, but that's not your loved one's goal. He or she is in pain—even though you may not see any signs of the pain.
- Migraine rarely is the cause of family problems. Most often it just makes existing problems obvious, or makes them worse.
- If you feel that a family member may be wanting to get out of chores or avoid family activities and uses migraines as a convenient excuse, don't stew about your feelings or bring them up in the middle of a fight. Schedule a time to talk about your feelings calmly and nonjudgmentally. Open communication is essential in a family affected by migraine.
- Your family is not alone in being disrupted by migraine. Every family with a migraineur faces the same issues. You will find great comfort in attending a headache support group.
- Get help if your family can't resolve migraine-related problems. See a family therapist who is experienced in dealing with people in chronic pain. And go before problems become critical—don't wait until your family has collapsed under the strain.

CHAPTER 27

Migraine at the Office

"There's a receptionist in my office who has migraines and has to go home frequently. The others hate her guts because they have to cover for her."

When it comes to dealing with an employee who has migraine, many companies are completely unprepared. Lacking a clear policy on how to handle sudden or frequent absences, the office may take a haphazard approach, pulling people off their own jobs to cover another's. In such a chaotic situation it's easy to understand why people would get angry at a co-worker with migraine. But the fault really does not lie with the migraineur, who didn't get sick on purpose and who would far rather be working than ill; instead, it lies with the employer, who has failed to adapt the office routine to incorporate the reality of migraine.

Most businesses ignore the needs of the millions of American workers with migraine. Millions of workdays are lost each year because of migraine, at a cost to the economy of billions of dollars. But an even larger sum is lost each year in unemployment and underemployment of migraineurs, who want to work but who can't find employers willing to hire them or to create schedules flexible enough to accommodate the needs of their condition.

Lack of knowledge about migraine among employers is a major obstacle for migraineurs in the work force. Although legal and social forces are at work to make employers more sensitive to the needs of people with disabilities, migraineurs so far have not seen many changes. They remain a silent and hidden group within the work force, unwilling to draw much attention to themselves and thereby risk their livelihoods.

TO DISCLOSE OR NOT TO DISCLOSE?

"Too many of us have spent endless, counterproductive energy denying to the world through our smiling faces and other disguises—especially to our nonheadache family, co-workers, employers and friends. We can't expect others to take migraine seriously if we do not."

To protect their jobs many migraineurs choose to hide their condition—or even to lie about it outright—when they apply for a job. Once hired, they often drag themselves to work during all but the worst migraine attacks and try to pretend nothing is wrong. When going to work is absolutely impossible, they make excuses or claim other health problems. Most admit that they can't work at peak efficiency with a migraine, yet they fear asking for the help and support they need from employers.

Should migraineurs disclose their illness to a prospective employer? In the past the answer often was not a matter of choice, since employers often used job application forms and interviews to ask discreet—and sometimes not-so-discreet—questions about a candidate's health status. The employer's aim was twofold: to weed out what would be considered possible drags on productivity, and to protect the employee health-insurance plan from a possible source of excessively high claims.

With passage of the 1990 Americans with Disabilities Act (ADA), such questions by all but the smallest employers now are prohibited. The ADA prohibits employers from discriminating against qualified people with obvious or hidden disabilities if they can perform the job with "reasonable accommodation" to their disability. (See Chapter 30.)

Under provisions of the ADA you do not have to answer questions about your health unless the questions are closely related to job tasks. Even if you volunteer information about migraine, the employer cannot use that information to deny employment unless the disability makes you substantially unqualified for the job.

The ADA's protections, when applied to migraine, will make it much easier for people to tell the truth about their condition if they choose. Still, many will continue to keep quiet until they've started the job, and even then to hold back as long as possible. Whatever the legal protections, they believe they risk losing their jobs if they are "found out."

HEALTH INSURANCE AND THE MIGRAINEUR

For many people with migraine finding and keeping a job is all-important because it represents the only affordable way of getting health-insurance coverage. Joining the employer's group plan often means you can qualify for better coverage at a cheaper rate, sometimes without even a waiting period for preexisting conditions.

The world of health insurance, however, is becoming increasingly complex. More than 60 percent of employers who offer health insurance now operate self-insurance plans. Although these plans are set up much like commercial insurance plans, the employer retains far more control over what the plan will and will not cover. In fact a recent case that reached the U.S. Supreme

Court permitted a self-insurance plan to reduce coverage for an employee with AIDS from a maximum lifetime benefit of $1 million to a maximum lifetime benefit of $5,000. Some fear the decision may be extended to others with chronic illnesses, including patients with migraine.

The changes that will result from national health care reform ultimately may make it easier for people with migraine to get, keep, and afford health-insurance coverage. Whatever form the changes take, however, they are almost certain to add new questions and complexities that migraineurs will have to learn to address.

SELF-EMPLOYMENT: AN EQUIVOCAL ANSWER

"Having migraine is economically devastating for families. If I didn't have my own business, I wouldn't be able to work."

Some people with migraine try to avoid the entire complex problem of educating the boss by going off on their own, either as a freelancer, an independent professional, or the owner of a small business.

If you are a professional with your own practice or your own business, you do have more choices than those who have to depend on an employer's goodwill about time off and insurance. You certainly have more control of lighting, smoking, and other environmental factors, and you can arrange for people to work in your place during migraine attacks.

Self-employment, however, has other pressures. Although there are undeniable payoffs in working for yourself, there is one major drawback: you don't earn any income if you can't work.

"I'm a therapist, and I have to cancel clients if I have a migraine. People don't get their money's worth if I can't focus. I will cancel in the middle of a day if a migraine comes on."

Self-employed people and small business owners today are increasingly faced with another problem: extremely high insurance costs. For people with chronic illnesses like migraine, disability insurance may be prohibitively expensive. Even health insurance may be priced out of reach, because small-group rates are based on the medical histories and claim records of the individuals being covered, not on a group average. National health care reform may change the picture somewhat, but it is not clear whether costs will go down, stay the same, or go up, especially in the short term.

ENLIGHTENED EMPLOYERS

"I worked at a local PBS station. They were wonderful. They knew I had migraines, and I missed one day a week at least. But I worked there almost ten years."

If you stay in the conventional work force and if you do decide to tell your "secret" to a prospective employer, be prepared for the worst: you may well find yourself out of a job or stalled in your career track. If you are lucky, however, you may discover that you're dealing with a sympathetic and fair-minded person who is willing to make the workplace accommodate your illness.

An employer who offers flexible scheduling and other options to a migraineur stands to benefit significantly in the long run. Studies indicate that the employer gains far more in productivity, loyalty, and job satisfaction than the company loses in sick time and insurance benefits for migraine.

In some particularly enlightened workplaces employers are making efforts to support better health for *all* their employees. For example, these employers often permit many categories of workers, not just people with migraine, to work a flexible schedule. Flexible schedules reduce stress for working parents, people taking classes at night, and anyone who doesn't fit the typical nine-to-five mold.

In addition, these employers often set up task forces to improve the work environment by modifying lighting, eliminating indoor pollutants, and substituting ergonomically designed office furniture for the typical uncomfortable, one-size-fits-all desks and chairs. Such changes help reduce environmental triggers for people with migraine and contribute to a healthier, more pleasant working environment for all.

Tips for Talking About Migraine to Employers

- **Take a hard look at yourself first.** Make a list of all the reasons you might want to tell your boss about your migraines. Don't hold back. Are you driven by a desire to be more genuine with your co-workers? Are you trying to educate your boss about migraine? Are you feeling self-pity or a desire for attention? Acknowledge all your motivations before you try to talk so you won't be sending any indirect messages.
- **Address the issue matter-of-factly.** You can certainly report to your employer that you have migraines that may sometimes incapacitate you. But it is probably inappropriate to stress the level of pain you experience or the troubles migraine has brought to your life.
- **Provide scientific information about migraine.** Tell your boss what you know about the causes of migraine. You may want to give him or her a brochure on migraine that presents the scientific facts in a readable way.
- **Tell your boss what you need in the way of support.** You can alleviate your boss's fear that your migraine condition will dominate the workplace by telling your boss specifically what you need to help you manage your

migraines in the workplace. For example, if perfume or smoke are triggers for you, let your boss know that your migraine attacks might be less frequent if you could work in a smoke-free and perfume-free environment. If you can ward off a migraine by taking medication and lying down at the first sign of a migraine, tell your boss.

- **Remember, not all bosses are equal.** Some employers will respond positively to your requests; some will assume you are being unreasonable. Keep in mind that when an employer doesn't respond positively, it does not mean you were wrong to disclose your illness or that you failed in your mission to educate.

CHAPTER 28

Migraine at School

"The first time I had a migraine I was in school. I lost my vision and ran into a wall. I was very upset and scared. After that I stayed at home in bed when I had migraine."

School years are supposed to be a child's start to a productive and fulfilled life. If those years are made miserable by recurrent headaches, however, a child may fall behind academically, socially, and in emotional development.

A primary goal for parents of school-age migraineurs should be to find the most effective migraine therapy for the child. When headaches are infrequent, children are less likely to lose ground or feel constant anxiety about their attacks.

The second important goal should be to help the child achieve the best possible school attendance record given the severity of the migraine disorder. Like all children your child really would prefer to be in school, sharing the activities of peers, learning new skills and growing in competence and confidence. Yet some children develop "school phobia" because of the fear, anguish, and humiliation that come with having an attack. You may inadvertently reinforce a child's phobia by keeping the child out of school longer than necessary in response to the child's obvious anxiety.

A KIND, EFFECTIVE ANTIDOTE TO SCHOOL PHOBIA

Migraine experts who work with children start with the premise that children want to fit in and be "normal," just like their peers who do not have headaches. A headache singles the child out, makes him or her appear "weird," "different," "weak," and "sickly." The sudden, uncontrollable vomiting that many children experience during migraine attacks humiliates them in front of peers and teachers. It also frightens them, because they cannot count on the comfort and safety of their familiar home, bed, and family when an attack comes during the school day.

Like adults who experience panic attacks in public places and then stop going outdoors for fear it will happen again, children can develop a phobia about school after a severe migraine attack there. Their anxiety builds each day as they dread the possible recurrence. Eventually the anxiety and stress will contribute to bringing on another attack—and a cycle of pain-dread-pain is established.

Parents can help break this cycle by acknowledging the child's fears while helping the child overcome them. Using a desensitization technique that is highly successful in treating phobias, the parent helps the child rebuild a sense of competence in the school environment.

Because desensitization decreases anxiety, it may decrease the frequency of migraine attacks in school, but that is not the primary goal of using the technique. The goal is to help the child maintain his or her inner motivation to go to school, despite the recurrent trauma of migraine.

A School Phobia Desensitization Plan

- Parent and child start by agreeing that it is important to go to school and talking about the good things that happen there.
- Parent and child reexamine the child's migraine experiences at school, with the goal of finding new ways for the child to cope.
- Parent and child agree on what the child can do when an attack starts coming on. The plan covers: who to tell; where the child will be taken when the headache hits; who will come for the child and when; and what the family will do for the child when they get back home.
- The child then begins going back to school for short, defined periods of time. The first day, for example, he or she may go back only for math or spelling period. One or two days later the stay is increased to two periods, then to a morning, then eventually to the entire day.
- When the next migraine occurs, parent and child reevaluate their plan of action and make changes if necessary.

SPECIAL NEEDS PROGRAMS

"School was difficult. I missed a lot. I had to leave and get home as soon as I felt a migraine coming on."

If parents deal firmly and lovingly with a child's fears of having a migraine attack in school, most children with migraine can keep up with their schoolwork, even though they miss some time now and then. But for children who have more severe forms of migraine disorder that do not respond well to treatment, absenteeism may threaten the child's academic progress.

Most school districts have special programs for children who are temporarily homebound because of illness. Typically, these programs are used for children who develop cancer and miss time because of the effects of treatment, or for children recovering from major illnesses or accidents.

You many have to work hard with your school principal to convince him or her to extend the homebound learning program to your child. "You have to break new ground to do it," said one parent of a child with severe migraine. "Many principals won't immediately see that children with severe migraine are seriously ill and warrant special accommodations."

If the principal is not well informed about migraine, he or she may believe you are coddling your child or reinforcing maladaptive responses to pain. And even if you are able to convince the principal, there often is a statutory limit on the number of days your child can receive homebound teaching during a school year. Homebound learning is a temporary solution, but it may be one worth investigating while your child's migraine crisis resolves itself or while you and your child's physician investigate other solutions to the problem of frequent absences.

If your child's school administration is cooperative, the homebound learning option can be used as part of a flexible scheduling plan that balances the need to motivate the child to return to the classroom with the imperative to help the child keep up with his or her studies when he or she is too ill to attend. In such an instance parent, child, teacher, and principal participate in making decisions about what is expected of the child and the parameters for when learning at home is appropriate. "Flexible scheduling is absolutely the best option for a child who has severe migraine," said one mother of a teenage migraineur.

LEARNING DISABILITIES AND MIGRAINE: IS THERE A LINK?

One of the myths about migraine in adults is that migraine is a sign of intelligence and special aptitude. Paradoxically, when migraine occurs in children, the more common myth is that migraine and learning disabilities are likely to coincide.

There is no convincing evidence to show that children with migraine are any different, statistically, from the rest of their peers, except in ways that are related specifically to migraine or that are attributable to the effects of chronic illness.

- Like adults with migraine, children with migraine may show mood disturbances, problems with thinking and concentration, or unusual behavior before a migraine develops. These changes are part of the biology of migraine—possibly linked to the neurotransmitter serotonin. Because some children get migraine equivalents instead of head pain (see Chapter 5), the symptoms aren't always clearly linked to migraine.
- Like adults with migraine, children may develop maladaptive responses to pain—sometimes called "secondary gain" (see Chapter 25). These maladaptive responses may make them seem less independent, less social, or less emotionally developed than their peers.
- Like adults with migraine, children with migraine may be medicated with drugs that alter their responses.
- Dietary factors, especially food sensitivities, are believed by some researchers to be a contributing factor in attention-deficit disorder and other learning disabilities. Because certain foods may be migraine triggers for a child, many people jump to the erroneous conclusion that migraine and learning disabilities have a common cause—when, in fact, neither can be said to be caused by foods.

Parents who are worried about their child's abilities can take comfort. Based on the current level of knowledge there is no reason to believe that children with migraine are either more or less likely to have organically based learning difficulties. In most cases they're just ordinary kids who happen to be headache-prone.

GUIDANCE COUNSELORS AND MIGRAINE

Teachers, principals, school nurses, and other school staff need a thorough orientation to migraine and its effects on children's lives. Another important but often-overlooked target for migraine education is the school guidance counselor.

Guidance counselors help children recognize their strengths and transform them into ambitions. A well-informed and migraine-sensitive guidance counselor can help children with migraine keep migraines in perspective as they begin planning for the future.

In dealing with the child who has migraine, a guidance counselor's motto might well be, "There are no unrealistic ambitions—only unrealistic time frames." For the child with a severe form of migraine disorder, for example, a counselor might suggest that the path to a bachelor's degree begin with one or two courses at a community college. For children whose migraine-related absences are affecting their grades, the guidance counselor might work with the child and parents to develop a desensitization program.

Above all the guidance counselor must remember that while the child's life may be affected by chronic pain and recurrent illness, the child has the hopes, dreams, and ambitions of any child the same age. The child will have the best chance of succeeding when these longings for normalcy are affirmed and when the child is helped to see possibilities for gaining more control over life.

HIGHER EDUCATION AND THE CHILD
WITH MIGRAINE

"I had to drop out one semester because I was tired and weak from migraines. I could have been finished a long time ago, but I took one class a semester because I was too worried about the load. I have only four classes left, but that will take me four more semesters."

Migraine is not necessarily the "glass ceiling" for a child's ambition to go on to college. Thousands of people with migraine successfully complete college—and graduate school—every year. If a child with migraine is motivated toward college, there is every chance that he or she will succeed.

Migraineurs sometimes report taking longer than usual to complete their degrees. Students may cut back their studies to half-time because the volume of reading required in a full course load triggers their headaches. Others find the stress of juggling multiple courses and deadlines too great. The college lifestyle itself—late hours, irregular eating and sleeping habits, high stress levels, possible use of alcohol or other drugs—is a minefield of potent migraine triggers.

Nonetheless most migraineurs choose to go through college in the typical sequence of four years. Many people who have experienced migraines throughout their lives, in fact, report that their college years were a time of relatively little migraine activity. Researchers have not turned up any scientific evidence to say how widespread this experience may be, nor is there any scientific explanation of why it should occur.

CHAPTER 29

Traveling with Migraine

"I once spent twelve hours in Memphis trying to get care for a terrible headache. The emergency room referred me to a drug hotline. My own sister's doctor kept me waiting for four hours."

Every migraineur has had the frustrating and disappointing experience of developing a headache while traveling. For many the headache comes the first morning after the airplane flight and robs them of the wonder and delight of the first day in a new place. Others have the humiliating and frightening experience of becoming ill en route. Trying to find a sympathetic doctor in a strange place, a pharmacy with your medications available, a quiet, dark place to recover—these are the most vivid memories some migraineurs have of their vacations and work-related travel.

Travel is a particularly common prelude to a severe migraine because it exposes migraineurs to many conditions that lead to attacks. Travel changes your normal schedule; it exposes you to different climates, altitudes, atmospheric conditions, and plants; it creates tremendous stresses as you try to get packed to leave, make travel connections on time, and squeeze every drop of zest out of each day that you're traveling.

SURVIVING A MIGRAINE WHILE TRAVELING

Unfortunately there's no way to guarantee you won't develop a headache when you travel. But there are many valuable precautions you can take that will lessen the chances you'll be caught helpless by a severe attack. For migraineurs pleasurable travel is not impossible, but it requires plenty of advance planning.

> "I used to take all my vacations in a camper—that was great! That way I always had a bed to crawl into if a headache came on."

The most important goal of all your advance preparation should be to lessen the stresses that accompany travel. Stress often makes people forget about their normal self-care habits— and for a person with migraine, as for someone with diabetes or any other chronic illness, keeping to a set schedule and an orderly routine can help make the difference between a manageable flare-up and a major crisis.

SELF-HELP FOR MIGRAINEURS ON THE GO

General

- Keep to your medication schedule! Many people forget about their medicines in the excitement and stress of the trip.

- At the first sign of a headache, *stop* and carry out your treatment plan. Don't wait until it is convenient. By that time you may already be in the most painful stage.
- If your migraines are linked to your menstrual cycle, plan your travel to avoid your most likely headache times.
- As much as possible, keep to your normal daily schedule— especially your usual hours for sleeping and eating. If you're in a different time zone, keep your watch on back-home time.
- Be especially cautious about travel to hot, humid areas. Many migraineurs report that heat (including overheated rooms) triggers particularly painful headaches.
- If you feel yourself getting a headache in an airport, train, or bus terminal, go to the Travelers Aid counter, or speak to the nearest security guard. Nearly all public terminals have a first-aid station or quiet room for travelers or employees.
- Ask your doctor about taking an antimotion sickness aid (Dramamine or the scopolamine patch) when you travel. Some migraineurs say it helps even though they do not experience a typical feeling of motion sickness.
- Avoid stressing your neck and shoulder muscles by carrying too-heavy shoulder bags or by sleeping in upright seats. Buy and use an inflatable pillow that supports your neck. For the baggage use a luggage cart.

Medical Care

- Carry your treatment plan and a letter from your doctor that states your diagnosis, the recommended emergency-room treatment, and any medications you *can't* take. In addition to the doctor's name and signature, the letter should include his or her DEA registration number. Tell the emergency-room admitting nurse that you will be willing to pay for a long-distance call to your doctor if needed.

- If you will be going abroad for an extended trip to an area where English is not spoken, see if you can arrange to have your doctor's instructions translated into the local language before you go. Your local classified telephone directory contains listings of translators in your area.
- Take twice as much medicine as you'll need for your time away. Carry half of it with you in hand luggage to allow for loss or damage to your checked baggage.
- Take written copies of your prescriptions with you.
- For international travel, be extra careful that your medicines are kept in properly labeled containers—customs officials will inspect them carefully.
- Some credit-card companies (such as American Express and VISA and MasterCard Gold) offer their customers worldwide assistance in finding English-speaking physicians. Keep the contact number with you. You can also contact the American embassy or consulate for assistance in finding a doctor.

Altitude

- If you will be flying long distances and/or staying in a region that is at a higher or lower altitude than home, talk to your doctor. Changes in altitude can affect the way medicines work in your body.

Stress

- Avoid the avoidable stressors. Ask your family and fellow travelers to help you with preparations for the trip and with the actual details of life on the road.
- Don't rush! Be sure to leave plenty of time to get to the airport or depot, or to your destination if you are driving.

Driving

- Avoid the factors in a long trip that stress you out. For example, if you dislike driving in city traffic but don't mind highway driving, arrange for a family member or companion to take the in-town driving shifts.
- Take breaks at least every two hours—more often if possible. Move around, drink water, do some relaxation exercises.
- Be sure you'll be traveling in an air-conditioned car.
- Keep your windshield and windows clean inside and out, to cut down on glare.
- Don't drive at night if you can avoid it, especially if you're susceptible to flickering lights.
- To cut down on the glare from sunlight or snow, wear a hat with a brim and sunglasses.

Airplane Travel

- Some people avoid "airplane headaches" by taking a single dose of over-the-counter antihistamines such as Sudafed a half hour before boarding the plan. (If you want to try this, talk to your doctor to make sure that you can safely take this medication and that your other medications are compatible.)
- If you're afraid to fly, find out if there are any special programs in your area to help people overcome this fear. The stress (and the alcohol some people use to blunt the fear) can trigger a headache.
- Drink plenty of water before, during, and after an airplane flight. Your body and nasal passages tend to become dehydrated in the dry pressurized cabin, and dehydration may trigger a headache. Do not drink alcohol while traveling—besides its power as a trigger for some people, it also makes you more dehydrated.

Hotels, Motels

- Ask to see your room before you accept it. If you notice any chemical smells (cleaning fluids, exterminator's chemicals, or smoke) that you suspect may cause you problems, go back to the desk and ask for another room.
- If you're sensitive to cigarette smoke, ask for a nonsmoking room. Many hotels and motels now designate such rooms.
- If the hotel or motel has a pool, sauna, or hot tub, ask for a room that isn't too near them. This way you'll put the maximum distance between you and their accompanying humidity, chemicals, and mildew.

CHAPTER 30

Health Insurance Issues

"Insurance companies are notoriously conservative when it comes to headaches. Insurance companies do not like to pay for this treatment."

Migraine patients often find themselves at a tremendous disadvantage in getting the benefits of their health-insurance coverage. Because migraine does not have a distinct diagnostic marker, insurers are skeptical of treatment related to headache. And because the area of interest is the brain, tests to rule out physical conditions that mimic migraine often are quite expensive.

Some people have no trouble receiving reimbursement for headache-related treatment. But insurance companies differ greatly in their practices. Getting appropriate reimbursement for headache-related diagnosis and treatment may require a significant investment of time on your part. You may have to appeal your claim through several levels of your insurance company, then take it to the state insurance commissioner. In the process your insurance company may try to drop you or raise your rates substantially.

The good news is that persistence often pays off. But many migraineurs resent the time, effort, and additional burden they face when trying to collect the insurance benefits they pay for.

TRADITIONAL HEALTH INSURANCE POLICIES

"Because I can only work part-time, I can't get health insurance. I can't afford it."

"I have coverage, but I pay for a lot of doctors, and I pay for psychotherapy myself."

For many longtime headache patients, especially those who are not employed or who are employed only part-time, standard health-insurance policies are prohibitively expensive. Many go without any insurance; some buy catastrophic insurance only, paying for day-to-day medications and treatments out of their own pockets.

Indemnity insurers typically reimburse you for a set percentage of your medical bills, leaving you to pay the copayment amount out of pocket. The insurer usually has a long list of excluded treatments and conditions, however, for which they will not pay a dime. Sometimes the exclusion is temporary, as when you change insurance plans and are asked to wait a certain number of months before submitting claims for conditions you had before. In more and more cases preexisting conditions are permanently excluded from coverage. Some plans also refuse to pay for psychotherapy, biofeedback, and other common adjunctive therapies used in migraine.

Migraine patients often are surprised when claims that would be covered for other conditions are rejected solely because they are for headache diagnosis and treatment. Most commonly the rejected claims are for diagnostic testing (such as MRI imaging) when accompanied by a headache diagnosis. In some cases insurers may also reject claims for medications, lab tests, and even office visits.

For headache patients, not having an MRI when headaches suddenly worsen or change patterns can be dangerous. The MRI may turn up a correctable physical problem, such as an aneurysm, that can be life threatening if left untreated. Many physicians believe an MRI or CT study is an essential first step in confirming a diagnosis of migraine for some patients.

If your claim is rejected or precertification (approval in advance for a procedure) is denied just because the procedure was headache related, appeal the decision using the insurer's in-house appeals process. Claims adjusters are taught to use the strictest interpretation of the rules when a claim is first evaluated; for this reason many appeals are won. Support your appeal with a letter from your physician explaining the importance of the procedure, test, medication, or treatment. Your physician usually will be happy to give you such a letter.

If your insurance company still refuses to pay your claim, or drops you from your plan, write to your state's insurance commissioner. It is important not to passively accept the insurance company's refusal to give you access to the treatment you need. Unfortunately, many insurance companies have to be prodded repeatedly before they change their reimbursement standards to reflect current medical practice for a condition.

HEADACHE CARE IN HMOs

Many migraine patients now get their health care in a health maintenance organization (HMO), preferred-provider organization (PPO), independent practice association (IPA), or other nontraditional insurance program. These plans try to provide health care at a lower cost by working with closed panels of doctors and a limited number of locations. Usually you select a primary-care physician who becomes the "gatekeeper," directing you to specialists or other caregivers when he or she thinks you can benefit from them.

Most HMOs and similar plans provide excellent medical care. When it comes to migraine treatment, however, your satisfaction largely depends on your primary-care physician's attitude. If he or she has an up-to-date understanding of migraine and is interested in working with you to find appropriate treatment, you may find it easy to get appropriate diagnostic tests and medications as well as needed referrals to specialists within the system.

If your primary-care physician seems uninterested in working with you to control your headaches, you may need to switch physicians. Most plans allow you to change primary-care physicians whenever you want.

If you have seen your HMO's neurologist and still haven't found a treatment plan that works, you may be able to convince your HMO to pay for visits to an outside headache specialist. Start the process by talking about your situation with your primary-care physician. Give him or her the name of the outside headache specialist you want to see. To bolster your claim that this level of care is necessary, use your headache diary (see Chapter 10) to document the frequency and severity of your pain.

Don't be shy in pressing your case with the HMO's bureaucracy. They collect your premium each month with the assurance that they can provide all your medical care. You are simply asking them to make good on their commitment to you.

MEDICARE AND MEDICAID

"I'm on disability—Medicare—and they now won't pay for self-injected DHE shots at home. Now I have to go to the emergency room, at five hundred dollars a shot."

For some migraine patients whose headaches are not controlled by current treatments, applying for Social Security disability or state assistance benefits is a way to solve two problems at once. First, the disability income helps keep the household afloat when work is impossible; and second, being designated as disabled makes you eligible for federal and state health-insurance coverage through Medicare and Medicaid.

Medicare and Medicaid are enormously complex health-care systems, expensive to operate and cumbersome to administer. Because of this complex structure Medicare personnel may make what seem like irrational decisions about what to pay and what to deny. It may seem utterly unbelievable, for example, that Medicare would deny a person autoinjectable DHE when a self-administered shot would cost so much less than an emergency-room visit to get the same drug. But given the way the regulations governing payment are written, such irrational-seeming policies abound.

Like private insurers Medicare has appeal procedures for denied claims. Depending on your doctor's status as a Medicare provider, the responsibility may fall to you to appeal the denial. Appeals move slowly and are less likely to succeed in the Medicare system than with a private insurer.

If you can afford private insurance supplementary to Medicare, part of the costs that Medicare doesn't pay may be absorbed by this insurer. Coverage and costs vary widely on Medicare supplement policies, so it's a good idea to shop around.

TAKING CHARGE OF YOUR INSURANCE

The practices of insurance companies in handling claims for headache treatment are vastly inconsistent and often medically indefensible. For this reason migraine patients often are successful in appealing denials of their insurance claims. But in many cases you must decide whether the battle for reimbursement is worth the time and energy it will take to carry it through.

What matters most is that you shouldn't put off critical medical tests, such as a diagnostic MRI, on the basis of cost alone. If cost is a problem, talk about it frankly with your physician. He or she may be able to suggest alternative ways to cover the costs (such as a hospital-sponsored medical line of credit or a facility that sponsors reduced-cost testing for patients who cannot afford to pay). Or your physician may be willing to help you get an expedited hearing from your insurance company because of the pressing medical need.

Tips for Dealing with Health-Insurance Issues

- Be persistent about getting specialized care for your headaches in an HMO. HMOs usually have neurologists or other specialists who can help when your primary-care doctor has done all he or she can. Many HMOs also will refer you outside if you make a good enough case for it.
- If your health-insurance company denies a claim for headache care, don't hesitate to appeal if the claim would have been paid for another illness. All insurers have an appeals process, and many appeals are won.
- If you don't get satisfaction from your insurer, make an appeal to your state's insurance commissioner.
- Contact your state or national legislators and let them know about your experiences.

CHAPTER 31

Society and Migraine

Just as there is no magic pill that will make migraine disorder disappear, there is no magic way to make society understand what it means to live with migraine. Society largely ignores the pain and anguish caused by migraine, despite an enormous number of people who experience that pain and intimately know that anguish.

THE IMPORTANCE OF VISIBILITY

"We need to let go of the mechanisms at work deep within our psyches that tap our guilt, shame, and embarrassment. We need to tell others that we do have migraine—to enable others with migraine to speak out also."

Marcia Seawell,
Rocky Mountain Headache
Association

Many migraineurs are extraordinarily capable of keeping the severity of their headaches hidden. Susan, for example, is a fifty-two-year-old woman who has had severe migraine headaches at least twice a month her entire adult life. Yet one of her closest friends, on learning that she was being interviewed for this book, was astonished to find out that Susan's headaches caused nausea and vomiting and could prostrate her for a day. "I have never known Susan to have even a little headache!" said the friend.

Migraineurs keep themselves together in public so that they won't risk the scorn of the non–headache-prone world. But in doing so they lose the greatest weapon they can have in fighting for greater understanding—visibility. It's much easier to ignore something you can't see. And on the other hand it is much easier to care about a problem if it is wearing a familiar face.

It takes tremendous courage and inner strength to be willing to say, "I'm ill—I'm having a migraine attack."

Letting others in on the secret of your pain will not always have a happy ending. But the risk may be worth the ultimate benefit, since that's how people learn best: one-on-one and face-to-face. No statistical summary, no article by a physician, no book on migraine, can match the good you can do by giving an honest account of your experiences with migraine.

FIGHTING FOR YOUR RIGHTS

"Never underestimate the power of a person with migraine headaches!"

Education is a slow process. In the interim, migraine patients may have to become very assertive to win rights more easily granted to people with other medical conditions.

Just as you may have to fight your insurance company to obtain fair reimbursement for medical expenses, you may also have to fight the state or federal government if you become so disabled by migraine that you cannot work. Programs like Social

Security disability insurance were created to provide a safety net when a working person becomes disabled. But for migraineurs the invisible handicap often means that the safety net disappears.

Many lawyers and physicians discourage migraine patients from applying for disability benefits. They know how hard it is to prove to a hearing examiner that headache can make someone unable to work. Ultimately, however, the choice is yours. If you persist, you may win. Two recent cases show it can be done: in Missouri a cluster-headache patient won state assistance benefits; and in California a migraine patient pleaded her appeal without the help of a lawyer and was granted Social Security disability benefits.

THE AMERICANS WITH DISABILITIES ACT: A MEANS OF ACHIEVING FAIRNESS

"Over time I went from being a highly successful over-achiever with an invisible disability to a mostly disabled person with a very visible handicap—pain."

As anyone who has experienced a severe migraine attack knows, a migraine is utterly disabling while it is going on—and often for some time before and after the head pain. Migraine can affect thinking, speech, motor skills, coordination, and other activities. The aura phase may interfere with vision and perception. The head pain and nausea usually make it impossible for the person to continue working or carrying out simple activities of daily living.

The problem however, is that migraine, like migraineurs themselves, remains largely invisible. There is no physical indicator of the intense pain and disability the migraineur experiences. And that leaves migraineurs at the mercy of others' empathy—a sometime prospect at best.

No one's rights and dignity should be left to the whim of individuals. It was for this very reason that the U.S. Congress in

1990 passed a sweeping new law called the Americans with Disabilities Act (ADA). This law, which has been phased in over several years, guarantees people with disabilities equal opportunity in jobs and in public accommodations (that is, any establishments that serve the public, such as hotels, restaurants, hospitals, physicians' offices, et cetera).

Under the ADA, people with disabilities no longer are given their rights only when dealing with an enlightened employer or shopkeeper. The law requires all employers over a certain size to make "reasonable accommodations" to keep workers with disabilities on the job. For people with physical handicaps such as deafness, blindness, or inability to walk or move, these accommodations may include special chairs or equipment, sign interpreters or readers, and adaptations of the physical plant such as curb cuts and Braille signs in elevators.

Exactly how the ADA applies to people with invisible disabilities such as migraine will be worked out over the next few years, probably in the courts. It might well be possible, for example, to negotiate a flexible schedule, rest arrangements, and special lighting or environmental conditions with an employer as a reasonable accommodation to a migraineur's needs. It might also be possible to encourage emergency rooms to set aside a quiet, dark place for migraineurs to wait for treatment as a reasonable accommodation in public accommodations.

One fact is certain, however: migraineurs do fall under the ADA's definitions of disability. As the case law based on the ADA develops, migraineurs are likely to see precedents set that they can apply to their own situations. The goal is not lawsuits, but fairness.

The ADA has been a powerful tool to educate many people about the needs and abilities of people with obvious disabilities. Migraineurs may soon be exploring ways in which the ADA can become an education tool on their behalf as well.

EDUCATION: THE NUMBER ONE TASK

During the past few years, and particularly since the founding of headache-patient groups such as the American Council for Headache Education (ACHE—see "Resources" at the end of this book), the American public has become much more aware of migraine as a real illness. Newspapers and magazines report on new discoveries. Even *People* magazine, which passes through the hands of millions of readers, has prominently featured stories on headache types and treatments.

Physicians, too, have become more aware of new developments in our understanding of migraine. Once it was unusual to find a family doctor who knew that migraine requires specialized treatment; today more and more are trying their patients on beta blockers and other preventive drugs as first-line treatment, rather than merely writing a prescription for a painkiller.

Much is changing—but much remains to be changed. The key to bringing about those changes lies in *asking for them.* Headache specialists nationwide are working with ACHE's 3,000 members to make sure the headache patient's voice is heard.

You, as a person who has experienced migraine, have a critical role to play in the future of migraine treatment. It is your task to educate your fellow citizens by standing up and letting them see and hear you. In numbers migraineurs have the power to see that headache receives priority in research and outreach.

It may feel unfair to you that, on top of your migraines, the task falls to you of educating family, friends, co-workers, school officials, insurance providers, and anyone else with whom you come in contact. Yes, it is an added burden. But in the long run your family, your children, and generations of migraineurs to come will thank you for your bravery and your foresight in stepping forward at this critical juncture.

Your greatest contribution to society, however, is your commitment to your own well-being. If you can learn to view your migraines as episodes in a chronic recurrent illness, and find ways to take good care of yourself, you will truly be a migraine survivor.

Resources

THE AMERICAN ASSOCIATION FOR THE STUDY OF HEADACHE (AASH)

Founded in 1959 during a meeting of the American Medical Association (AMA), AASH seeks to bring together physicians from different specialties to share concepts and developments about headache. Today AASH is the leading professional society of nearly 1,000 physicians and other health-care providers dedicated to headache treatment and research.

AASH provides physicians with opportunities to learn about ongoing research on headaches and about the clinical management of headache disorders. These opportunities include an annual scientific meeting, professional training courses, and a scientific journal, *Headache,* published ten times a year.

Through involvement in the American Council for Headache

Education (ACHE), an organization founded by AASH members, AASH physicians disseminate the results of their research and clinical experience to benefit the millions of Americans who experience headache in any of its forms. AASH also provides physicians with patient education resources developed in cooperation with the ACHE. For information about membership in AASH, contact the association's executive offices at (609) 845-0322.

THE AMERICAN COUNCIL FOR HEADACHE EDUCATION (ACHE)

The American Council for Headache Education (ACHE) is a nonprofit organization dedicated to public education, scientific research, and advocacy for people who experience headaches. Founded in 1990, ACHE is a partnership between the professionals of the American Association for the Study of Headache (AASH) and people with headache and their families.

Speaking for its more than six thousand members, ACHE works to build bridges between headache patients and the healthcare community, insurance companies, legislators, the media, and the general public. Through public education about headache and its impact on society, ACHE works to create a climate for better understanding and increased scientific research to benefit people with headache.

Membership is open to anyone interested in the problem of headache. ACHE members receive the following privileges:

- A quarterly newsletter containing the latest information on treatment of the major forms of severe headache as well as practical guidance on coping with chronic head pain. It also reports on ACHE activities, legislative developments, and research support. The newsletter features interviews with headache patients and a column that answers readers' questions.

- Educational brochures on the major types of headache and options for treatment, including medication and nondrug therapies.
- Advance information on free public education seminars.
- Listing of current AASH members for physician referral.
- An opportunity to participate in forming local community headache support groups to share common concerns and challenges.
- An opportunity to join with thousands of patients and medical experts in educating employers, the health-insurance industry, and legislative leaders involved in funding of health care and research.
- Electronic support network. ACHE has gone on-line, providing expanded access to headache information and support via Prodigy, CompuServe, America Online, and the Internet.

For further information on ACHE, call

1-800-255-ACHE

or write to

American Council for Headache Education
875 Kings Highway, Suite 200
Woodbury, NJ 08096

HEADACHE SUPPORT GROUPS

Headache support groups are an important vehicle for people with headache to come together, share common problems and solutions, and discover that they are not alone.

ACHE has established a growing network of headache support groups. Contact with other headache sufferers offers a unique opportunity to share problems in confidence and to develop mutual strategies for problem solving and coping.

For information on joining an ACHE support group in your area, call ACHE at: 1-800-255-ACHE.

For Further Reading

The Headache Book: Effective Treatments to Prevent Headaches and Relieve Pain. Seymour Solomon, M.D., and Steven Fraccaro (Mount Vernon, New York: Consumer Reports Books, 1991); 191 pages.

Headache Relief: A Comprehensive, Up-to-Date, Medically Proven Program That Can Control and Ease Headache Pain. Alan M. Rapoport, M.D., and Fred D. Sheftell, M.D. (New York: Simon and Schuster, 1990); 288 pages.

Help for Headaches: A Guide to Understanding Their Causes and Finding the Best Methods of Treatment. Joel R. Saper, M.D. (New York: Warner Books, 1987); 234 pages.

Index